Discharge Planning for Home Health Care

A MULTIDISCIPLINARY APPROACH

AF732462

Barbara Stover Gingerich, RN, MS
Editor, *Journal of Home Health Care Practice*

Administrative Director
Rehabilitation/Community Health Services Division
St. Joseph Hospital
Lancaster, Pennsylvania

Partner
Advantage Health Care Management Resources
York, Pennsylavnia

Deborah Anne Ondeck, RN, BS
Editor, *Journal of Home Health Care Practice*

Manager
Home Health and Hospice Services
St. Joseph Hospital
Lancaster, Pennsylvania

Partner
Advantage Health Care Management Resources
York, Pennsylvania

AN ASPEN PUBLICATION®
Aspen Publishers, Inc.
Gaithersburg, Maryland
1994

Library of Congress Cataloging-in-Publication Data

Gingerich, Barbara Stover.
Discharge planning for home health care : a multidisciplinary approach / Barbara Stover Gingerich, Deborah Anne Ondeck.
p. cm.
Includes bibliographical references and index.
ISBN: 0-8342-0572-6
1. Home care services. 2. Hospitals—After care—Planning.
3. Hospitals—Admission and discharge. I. Ondeck, Deborah Anne.
II. Title
RA973.G56 1994
362.1'4—dc20
93-46662
CIP

Copyright © 1994 by Aspen Publishers, Inc.
All rights reserved.

Aspen Publishers, Inc., encourages and permits the photocopying of small portions of this work for personal or internal use. Written permission is not required for limited use. This consent does not extend to other kinds of copying, such as copying for general distribution, for advertising or promotional purposes, for creating new collective works, or for resale. For information, address Aspen Publishers, Inc., Permissions Department, 200 Orchard Ridge Drive, Suite 200, Gaithersburg, Maryland 20878.

Editorial Resources: Ruth Bloom

Library of Congress Catalog Card Number: 93-46662
ISBN: 0-8342-0572-6

Printed in the United States of America

1 2 3 4 5

We dedicate this manual
to our spouses:
Robert A. Gingerich
Michael G. Ondeck
and our children:
Jade Ann Gingerich
Wade A. Gingerich
Christopher M. Ondeck

◆ Table of Contents ◆

INSERT

TAB

◆ Introduction ◆

Discharge planning is recognized as a basic component of the patient's hospitalization. Regulations dating back to 1965 have had as their primary purpose in passage access to care, cost of care, or concern for quality and standard of care. The major regulatory acts that affect discharge planning are outlined in Table I–1. In addition to these, the introduction of the terms *diagnosis-related groups* and *average length of stay* into the health care provider's daily vocabulary caused hospital administrators to scurry to delegate the responsibility for development and implementation of a comprehensive systemwide discharge plan.

Task forces were formed, policies and procedures written, and utilization review departments founded, as discharge planning took on a new meaning and emphasis throughout all health care settings. These task forces had a similar goal: to develop a systematic discharge plan that would provide early assessment of patient and family needs along with consistent ongoing planning for that soon-to-occur event, the discharge.

Concurrently, because of the increase in the number of patients who were being discharged quicker and sicker, there was a correlative rise in home health care providers. The emergence of home care is described in detail in Chapter 1.

Table I–1 Regulatory Impacts on Discharge Planning

Date	*Origin*	*Source*	*Focus*	*Effect/Discharge Planning (DP) Task*
1951	Joint Commission on Accreditation of Healthcare Organizations	Private	Continuity of care	Coordination of medical, nursing, and social discharge plans; liaison with community health care providers DP task: Team approach to a written plan with documented implementation
1965	Medicare Title XVIII	Federal	Care access	Decreased financial barriers to health care; established benefits via Social Security Act for hospital, home health, and nursing home care DP task: Understand regulations, determine services needed, assist in placement and screening
1965	Medicaid Title XIX	State/federal	Care access	Provided care to categorically needy through facilities that meet Medicaid conditions of participation for quality of care DP task: Understand local Medicaid program and financial and social eligibility requirements; assist with enrollment and appropriate discharge placement via screening
1972	Professional Standards Review Organization (PSRO)	Federal: Department of Health, Education and Welfare; Private: PSRO	Cost	Appropriateness and quality of care provided are evaluated in relationship to geographic standards DP task: Develop close working relationship with PSRO; document early discharge planning; certify level of care needed
1974	Public Laws	Federal	Cost	Established state health planning and development agencies, state health coordinating councils, and regional

Table I–1 continued

Date	*Origin*	*Source*	*Focus*	*Effect/Discharge Planning (DP) Task*
				health system agencies to review facility and service plans DP task: Articulate first-year and 5-year discharge plan; statistic summation and reporting for inclusion in state health plan
1975	Social Security Act	Federal/state	Cost	Mandated citizen participation and review to increase provision of care to categorically needy DP task: Know of Title XX services available; convey to state needs for new programs as identified
1983	Diagnosis-Related Groups (DRGs)	Federal	Cost	Designated lump sum payment for hospital providers based on diagnosis of patients DP task: Early screening and implementation of discharge planning; knowledge of placement criteria and community resources
1992	Resource-Based Relative Value Scale (RBRVS)	Federal	Cost	Overhauls physician Medicare payments and reduces same to physicians in teaching or university hospitals; does not consider severity of illness of patient DP task: Know effect on physicians in subspeciality and early intervention to encourage physician groups to participate in early discharge planning

This combination of regulatory issues seeking quality cost-effective care, the increased acuity of the discharged patient, and home care's readiness to meet the growing need for highly trained and competent health professionals within the community led to the need for incorporation and enhancement of the home care coordination link in the discharge planning process. This manual provides a comprehensive, step-by-step approach to organizational discharge planning.

Barbara Stover Gingerich
Deborah Anne Ondeck

◆ Acknowledgments ◆

We extend our thanks to those health care professionals who helped us as we separately pursued the development of a discharge planning model in West Virginia, Ohio, and Pennsylvania during 1984 to 1988 and also those health care professionals who have assisted us in this joint endeavor.

To our families and friends who have encouraged us and supported us through the development of this manual, we give our thanks and love.

INSERT

TAB

◆ Chapter 1 ◆

Overview

HISTORICAL PERSPECTIVE ON DISCHARGE PLANNING

From a historical perspective, discharge planning, or planning for continuity of care, has always been a basic part of the patient's hospitalization course. Several of the five basic questions—when, who, where, what, and why—have undergone significant changes from the 1950s to the 1990s.

First, the *when* question is the time frame for development and implementation of the discharge plan. The average length of stay (ALOS) has been shortened from the 1950s through the 1980s, with an expectation that there will be an ongoing decrease in ALOS throughout the 1990s.

Second, the *who* question focuses on the major contributors to the discharge plan. Although ALOS has been shortened, the range of contributors has expanded. The major contributors to the discharge plan in the 1950s included the nurse, social worker, and physician, but today this list has become multifaceted, and the team has as its central figure the patient and his or her support system.

Third, the *where* question is the setting. Where is discharge planning being done? This arena has also seen expanded emphasis. Today not only is discharge planning an important aspect of care in the medical/surgical units of acute care facilities, but there is also an increasing emphasis on the progressive care, intensive care, and acute care specialty units. The discharge planning arenas of the 1990s have continued to expand and now include primary care and outpatient clinics and the emergency departments of acute care hospitals as well as outpatient day surgery units and freestanding surgery centers. The setting continues to expand beyond acute care and now includes rehabilitation centers, Veterans Administration and mental health facilities, skilled nursing and personal care homes, surgery centers, and chemical detoxification programs.

The *what* aspect of discharge planning is the ongoing goal to develop a comprehensive, realistic, and affordable postdischarge plan that meets the individual's needs. Although the essence of discharge planning remains unchanged, in actuality the magnitude of the plan has increased. For example, what health care provider of the 1950s would have included home ventilator care in a patient's discharge plan?

These facts combined—the shortened time frame, the expanded team, the enlarged setting, and the magnitude of today's discharge plan—form the basis of the need for an institutionwide planned approach to the *why*.

Why do discharge planning? A need analysis approach to the four question areas above has had a drastic impact on the why question of discharge planning. Coordinated discharge planning is done to:

- provide ongoing quality care to patients
- ensure the appropriate care setting
- decrease ALOS
- increase patient compliance
- enhance reimbursement
- meet federal and state regulations
- utilize cost-efficient care modes
- meet comprehensive needs of patients and families
- ease patient/family fears and insecurities
- decrease the discharging facility's risk and liability
- improve the individual's quality of life
- meet Joint Commission on Accreditation of Healthcare Organizations standards
- comply with American Hospital Association guidelines
- ensure access to community health care systems and resources
- lower readmission rates
- decrease posthospitalization complications

The list goes on ad infinitum and varies in priority based upon the current conditions that exist within any health care system. Your list should be customized to your health care setting to acquire the needed administrative support. This support is necessary to the development and implementation of any discharge plan.

One of the first steps in acquiring administrative support is to complete a needs assessment analysis that demonstrates the need for a formal discharge plan within your health care system. A needs assessment measures the state of discharge planning within an institution while identifying the causative factors connected to this state.

Exhibit 1–1 identifies 10 steps to conduct a needs assessment. Step 1 identifies our primary objective to be the development of a comprehensive hospital–home care coordination/discharge plan. Assessment tools have been included for your customization and use in conducting Steps 2 to 4 of this needs assessment. Exhibit 1–2 addresses Step 2, the identification and selection of data-gathering sources; these need to be assessed to gather the data. This list can be adapted to your specific situation.

Steps 2 and 3 can be completed with many types of assessment formats. Some examples include the following:

- agency/consumer group surveys (Exhibit 1–3)
- patient questionnaires (Exhibit 1–4)
- patient interviews (Exhibit 1–4)
- patient telephone surveys (Exhibit 1–4)
- computer search
- research
- public forums

In Step 5, the data obtained are summarized for the specific needs identified and are presented to administration in Step 6. Chapter 2 addresses the ongoing Steps 6 to 10 of this needs assessment and implementation process.

Exhibit 1–1 How To Conduct a Needs Assessment

Step 1: Identify and prioritize objectives
Step 2: Identify and select data-gathering sources
Step 3: Conduct assessment of current services
Step 4: Collect information
Step 5: Synthesize information
Step 6: Present information
Step 7: Develop the plan
Step 8: Implement the plan
Step 9: Evaluate the plan
Step 10: Revise the plan

Exhibit 1–2 Data Gathering Sources Identification Checklist

				Assessment Desired		
Resources	*Type of Location*	*Yes*	*No*	*Yes*	*No*	*Type*
Consumers	American Association of Retired Persons					
	Church					
	Social					
	Fraternal					
	Office of Aging					
	Adult protective services					
	Child protective services					
	Population at large					
Service providers	Hospitals: Utilization review/Quality improvement					
	Social services					
	Physicians					
	Nurse managers					
	Therapists					
	Rehabilitation centers: Vocational rehabilitation counselors					
	Discharge planners					
	Case managers					
	Long-term care settings: Social workers					
	Nursing staff					
	Administration					
	Insurance companies: Blue Cross/Blue Shield					

DISCHARGE PLANNING FOR HOME HEALTH CARE
Copyright © 1994, Aspen Publishers, Inc.

Exhibit 1–2 continued

Resources	*Type of Location*	*Yes*	*No*	*Assessment Desired* *Yes*	*Assessment Desired* *No*	*Type*
	Health maintenance organizations					
	Preferred provider organizations					
	Physician hospital organization					
	Medicare					
	Medicaid					
	Home care agencies: Intake coordinator					
	Clinical supervisor					
	Social workers					
Community resources	Library					
	Diagnosis-specific agencies: Chief executive officers					
	Caregivers					
	Computer files					
	Leaders: Government					
	Health care					
	Corporate					
	Social					
	Church					
	Union					
	Collegiate					
	Census data					
	Government departments: Health					
	Welfare					

Copyright © 1994, Aspen Publishers, Inc.

Exhibit 1–3 Agency/Consumer Group Needs Assessment

1. Name: ____________________

2. Phone Number: ____________________

3. Date of Initial Contact: ____________________

4. Was client recently hospitalized? Yes_____ No_____

   If yes, which hospital? ____________________

5. Did the hospital provide discharge planning? Yes_____ No_____

   If yes, by whom? Nurse only_____ Social Worker_____ Home Care Coordinator_____ Therapist_____ Physician_____ Other_____

6. State reason for contact (i.e., what is the problem): ____________________

   ____

7. Are you currently receiving services from a home care agency? Yes_____ No_____

   If yes, agency name ____________________

   Who contacted them for you? ____________________

   Do you know how to contact them? Yes_____ No_____

8. Would you like someone to contact you who can help arrange the care that you may be eligible for? Yes_____ No_____

9. Do you have a preference? No_____ Yes_____ (Specify) ____________________

   If no, ___Agency A___ is piloting a needs assessment and will be contacted regarding your need.

Note: Please call ___Agency A___ and ask for ___Jane Smith___ to relay the client information necessary.

DISCHARGE PLANNING FOR HOME HEALTH CARE
Copyright © 1994, Aspen Publishers, Inc.

Exhibit 1–4 Sample Patient Questionnaire (Telephone/Mail/Interview)

Name: (optional) ______________________________

Address: (optional) ______________________________

____

Hospital Admission Date: ______________________________

Hospital Discharge Date: ______________________________

Diagnosis: ______________________________

Home Care Provided? Yes_____ No_____

Other Follow-Up Care? Yes_____ No_____

If yes, please specify type: ______________________________

Did you have any problems at home with the following?

1. Ambulation: Yes_____ No_____ If yes, specify ______________________________
2. Stairs: Yes_____ No_____ If yes, specify ______________________________
3. Transfers: Yes_____ No_____ If yes, specify ______________________________
4. Bathing: Yes_____ No_____ If yes, specify ______________________________
5. Medications: Yes_____ No_____ If yes, specify ______________________________
6. Meal Preparation: Yes_____ No_____ If yes, specify ______________________________
7. Transportation: Yes_____ No_____ If yes, specify ______________________________

Were you rehospitalized? Yes_____ No_____ If yes, specify ______________________________

Which home care staff provided care for you?

- Nurse: Yes_____ No_____
- Nurse's Aide: Yes_____ No_____
- Physical Therapist: Yes_____ No_____
- Occupational Therapist: Yes_____ No_____
- Speech Therapist: Yes_____ No_____
- Social Worker: Yes_____ No_____
- Other: Yes_____ No_____ If yes, specify

Did you have need of any of the above staff who did not provide care to you? Yes_____ No_____
If yes, specify ______________________________

Any additional comments? ______________________________

____

Copyright © 1994, Aspen Publishers, Inc.

HOME CARE'S EMERGENCE AS A HEALTH CARE PROVIDER

With the advent of the first regulatory health care legislation in 1965, home health began to emerge as a dominant force in the health care field. The number of Medicare-certified home health agencies grew from 1,753 in 1967 to 6,902 in 1993 (Figure 1–1). Of these home health agencies, there was an increase of 1,116 percent in the hospital-based sector, from 133 in 1967 to 1,934 in 1993 (Figure 1–2).

Hospitals were motivated to develop their own hospital-based agencies to develop feeder sources for inpatient admissions and to provide cost-effective alternative care for non-reimbursed lengthy inpatient stays. The focus in home care went from the chronic long-term patient to the acute high-tech patient. As the patient mix within the home health care field changed, so did the volume of patients being seen as well as the number of visits required by each patient. Patient referrals escalated from 392,700 in 1967 to 1,600,200 in 1990 (Figure 1–3) with a correlative rise in visits from 8 million in 1967 to 100 million in 1991 (Figure 1–4).

Many of the discharge plans developed in the early to mid-1980s failed to incorporate, or incompletely incorporated, an important aspect of discharge planning: home care coordination. This manual recognizes this need and provides a comprehensive program for implementation of a home care coordinated discharge plan for use in acute care facilities and home health agencies. Ease of adaptation to a wide variety of health care settings has been considered in anticipation of the expanding discharge planning needs of the 1990s and beyond.

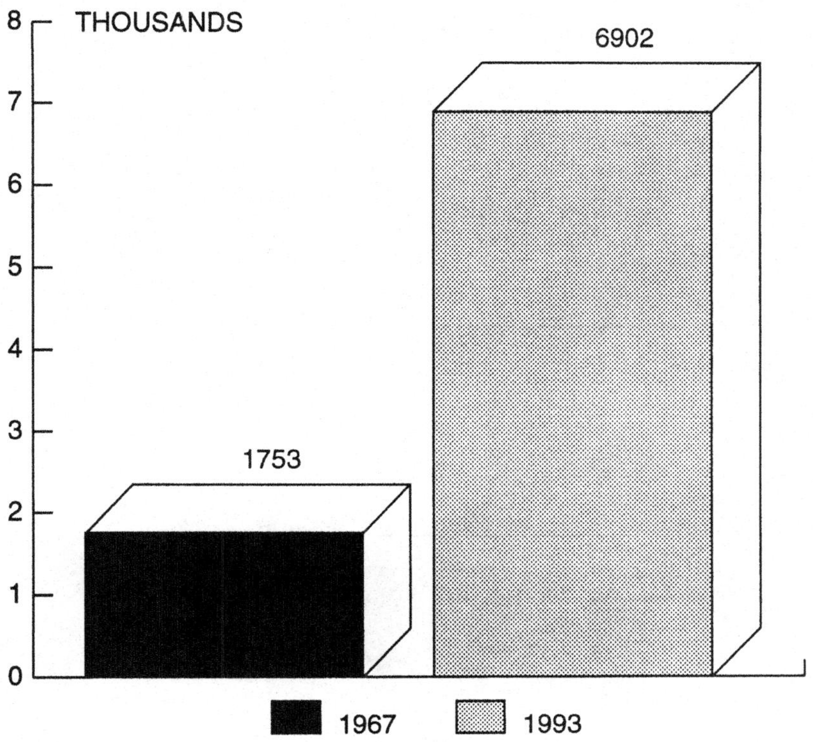

Figure 1–1 Total certified home health agencies.

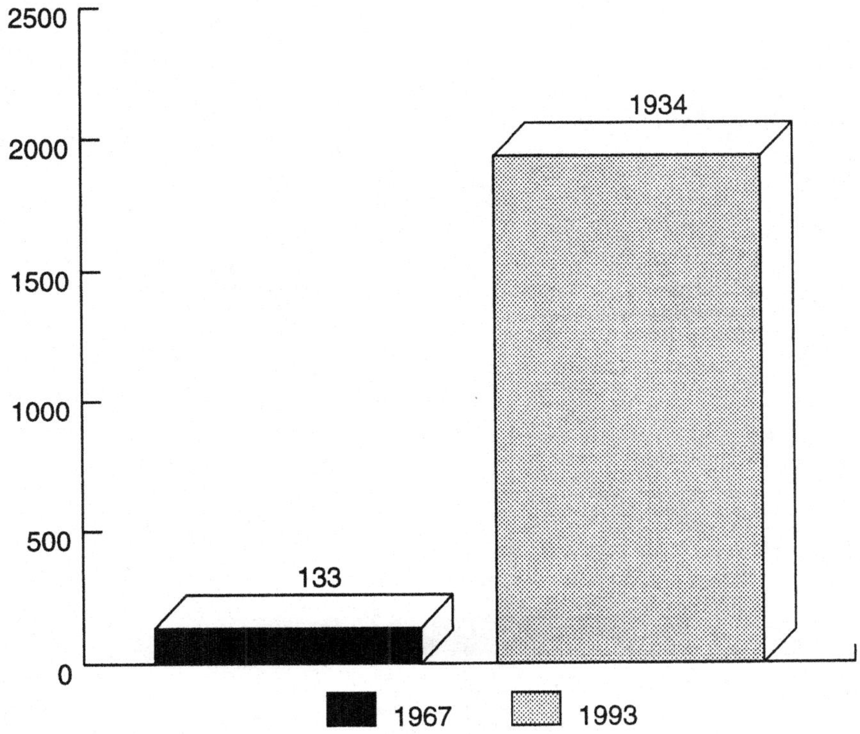

Figure 1–2 Hospital-based home health agencies.

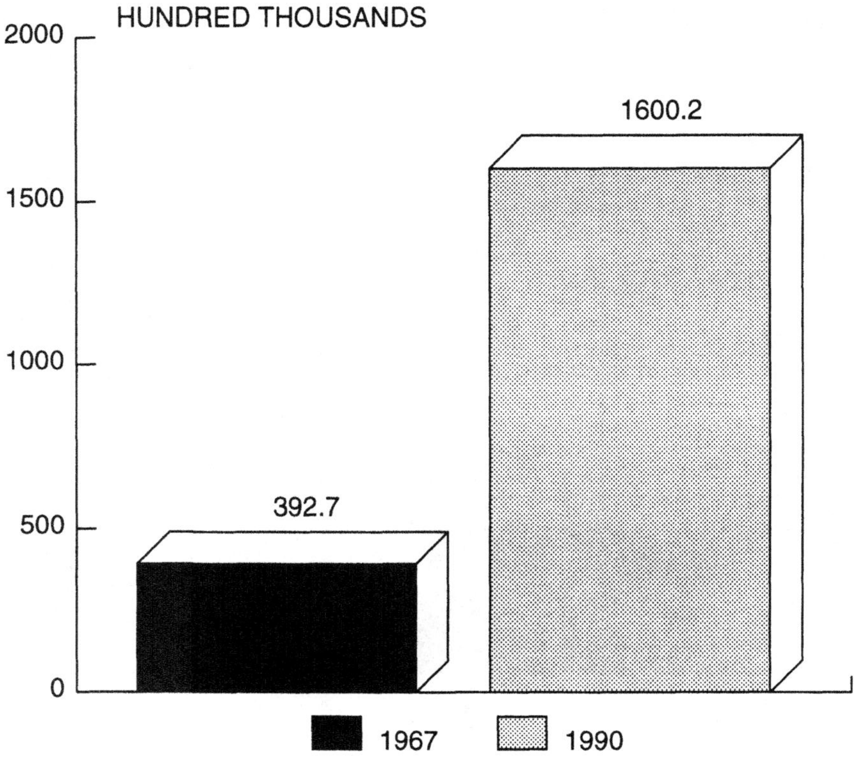

Figure 1–3 Patient referrals.

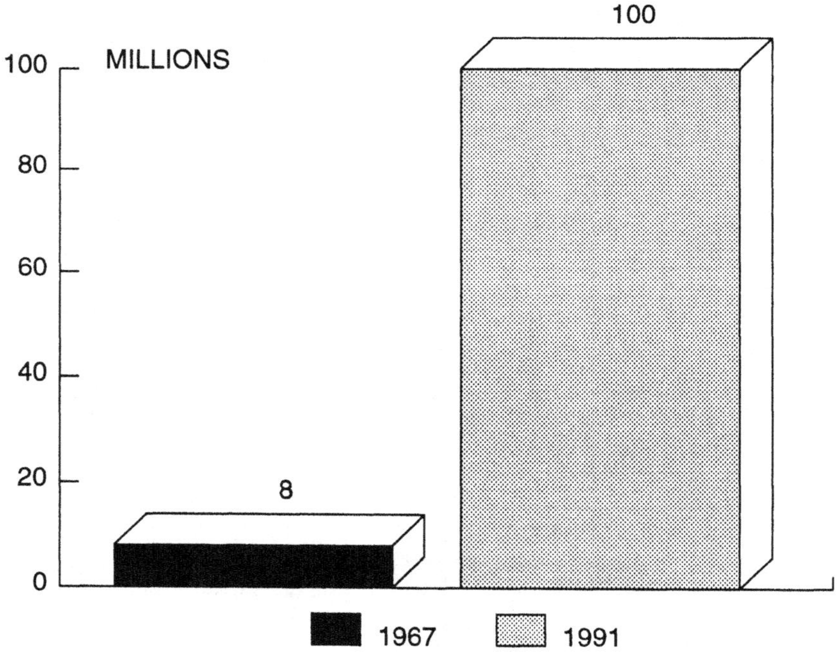

Figure 1–4 Home visits made.

◆ Chapter 2 ◆

The Hospital Discharge Plan

Once a concrete analysis of the community's resources and needs is available, internal networking should occur. The intent of this networking is to elicit widespread support for the establishment of a well-coordinated institutional discharge plan aimed at connecting patients with necessary resources in a timely, cost-effective manner. Usually at the heart of the discharge planning process is Social Services or Home Care Services. Internal networking begins when representatives from one or both of these departments present the gathered data supporting the need for a hospitalwide discharge plan to upper management. Broad-based administrative support is needed to obtain the widespread recognition and support required to develop this comprehensive plan. Internal networking continues to spread through informal communications which motivates disciplines involved in the individualized patient plan.

A Discharge Planning Task Force brings together the multidisciplinary team. Exhibit 2–1 explains the mission, objectives, composition, and agenda for the task force and completes the 10 steps listed in Chapter 1. Personality characteristics of task force members should include a willingness to be objective, an ability to offer and accept constructive criticism, an ability to work together as a team, an ability to focus with broad vision, an ability to resolve territoriality conflict issues, and a motivation to accomplish the objective. The facilitator should possess strong conflict management and communication skills. In any task force, you will find those who are resistant to change. How to counter this resistance and deal effectively with the change process is discussed in Chapter 8.

Exhibit 2–1 Discharge Planning Task Force

Mission: ABC Hospital's multidisciplinary task force is dedicated to providing all patients with a comprehensive discharge plan, including postdischarge referrals within the availability of our community's resources. We recognize our legal, moral, and ethical responsibility to our patients, institution, and community.

Objectives:
1. To identify current practices that delay discharge.
2. To reduce length of stay through implementation of a written discharge plan.
3. To develop interdepartmental collaboration toward individualized discharge plans.
4. To develop a comprehensive multidisciplinary methodology that evaluates all high-risk patients.
5. To incorporate patient rights and safety concerns into individualized postdischarge plans.
6. To promote continuity of care through provision of essential information.
7. To ensure utilization of appropriate health care settings based upon acuity levels.
8. To assist with the establishment of clinical pathways.

Members:

Hospital Board
Administration
Admissions/Pre-Admissions
Finance
Utilization Review
Home Care Services
Respiratory Therapy
Physical Therapy
Occupational Therapy
Quality Improvement
Pastoral Care
Medical Staff
Nursing
Social Services
Speech Therapy
Dietary

MEETINGS

Number	*Agenda*	*Follow-up*
1	Introduction by chairperson/facilitator Appointment of secretary Self-introduction of members, to include a brief statement of current involvement with discharge plan Round-table discussion of purpose, mission, objectives, and proposed time frames	All members to develop a list from their individual and departmental perspectives of existing problems with current discharge practices and possible resolutions (task force members are encouraged to elicit feedback from their departments)

DISCHARGE PLANNING FOR HOME HEALTH CARE
Copyright © 1994, Aspen Publishers, Inc.

Number	*Agenda*	*Follow-up*
2	Brainstorming session to identify and list current problems Systematic approach to development of plan, including: • screening of patients • discharge planning procedure for identified categories of patients • multidisciplinary roles/responsibilities • miscellaneous information • coordination of unit discharge planning meetings • evaluation of individualized plans	Interdepartmental meetings to focus on areas of territoriality, conflict, and compromise; ongoing documentation of plan development by chair-person
Final	Distribution of written hospital discharge plan to all members	Department meetings to review plan; implementation of plan (Step 8)
3 Months after imple-mentation	Plan evaluation (Step 9) Revision of plan as appropriate (Step 10)	Communication of plan's effectiveness and revisions

Discharge Planning for Home Health Care
Copyright © 1994, Aspen Publishers, Inc.

TERRITORIALITY

The issue of territoriality often arises as the discharge plan is committed to writing. The fear of loss of authority and power is often the basis of territoriality issues. This fear is grounded in the potential transfer of job roles and responsibilities to another discipline that will affect full-time equivalents and job security. Territoriality is often an issue between the social worker and the home care department's discharge planner. Unless it is addressed directly, the outcome of the task force could be hampered and become a source of frustration while inflexible members exhibit uncooperative behavior, antagonism, and destructive criticism. By avoiding the issue, areas of duplicity will continue to cost the institution lost time, money, and public image as patients and families are barraged with repeated questions and possibly incomplete discharge planning.

CONFLICT

At the root of any conflict there is disagreement, which results in anxiety and tension. One issue in the establishment of an organization's discharge plan is who approaches the patient first, the social worker or the home care discharge planner. When roles are completely dependent or completely independent, there is little room for conflict. As roles become more interdependent, however, the areas of conflict escalate.

Categories creating conflict are facts, methods, goals, and values. Placed from left to right, these form a conflict continuum that shows heightened conflict as the categories of disagreement advance to the right. To manage conflict, members of the discharge planning task force must trust themselves and others, must be committed to stay with the problem until it is resolved, and must communicate their thoughts and desires while actively listening. Table 2–1 explains problem-solving methods, and Exhibit 2–2 reflects the principles of problem solving. Exhibit 2–3 is a conflict area analysis work sheet. Much has been written about conflict management, and the reader is encouraged to explore this topic for a more in-depth understanding.

COMMUNICATION

The purpose of communication is to promote understanding between the sender and receiver of a message. It must be recognized that often the message sent is not the message received. Why? Barriers to communication are saboteurs lurking within both the sender and the receiver. Exhibit 2–4 lists barriers to communication and gives a diagram that illustrates how barriers inhibit understanding. Barrier busters used to enhance the communicative process can be found in Exhibit 2–5. Effective communication requires an active listener and an awareness of barriers and barrier busters by both parties.

Each task force member is an expert in his or her field. Brainstorming identifies strengths and weaknesses of your organization's current discharge planning process. The facilitator must emphasize the need for a team concept in the preparation and implementation of the overall discharge plan. It is imperative that each member recognize and value the education and capabilities of the other team members. Permitting dependent roles to continue to exist will do an injustice to your planning process. Team members need flexibility and permission to do their jobs without restraint. They must use time management techniques and take advantage of every available opportunity. They will be effective only if allowed to be independent in their area of expertise, but they must be considerate of the other members' roles and responsibilities. Once the team members realize that there is no need to feel threatened, they will be able to work together, like a precision machine, toward the ultimate goal of a comprehensive, timely, and individualized patient discharge plan.

The culmination of your Discharge Planning Task Force work may simulate the model discharge plan shown in Appendix 2–A. Sample tools that can be utilized by your institution are available in Chapters 3 through 7. These can be incorporated into your discharge plan.

FINAL STEPS

The hospital's discharge plan is now committed to writing. Undoubtedly, a few heated debates behind closed doors occurred, but it is hoped that those differences have been set aside with the finalization of the plan. This will minimize the number of patients who fall through the cracks. The new task at hand is for all members to educate their respective departments about the total plan.

Community resources should also be apprised of the changes in the plan and the resultant effects it may have on their agencies. As an example, consider the hospital's plan that prohibits outside home care agency personnel from doing their own coordination. The outside agency may feel threatened initially, but once the benefits are recognized the outside agency will be supportive of the hospital plan. It is suggested that a brief questionnaire (Exhibit 2–6) be sent to community referral agencies to help evaluate the plan's effectiveness. Should the comments indicate a need for revision, the task force can reconvene before the planned 3-month meeting for complete evaluation and revision. Of course, the patient questionnaire (Chapter 1) results will provide a valuable piece of information.

Central to the discharge planning in your hospital is the unit's weekly discharge planning meeting. A word of caution to overzealous participants: It is often easy to decide the fate of the absent patient based upon the diagnosis and minimal discussion time. We must avoid this pitfall of categorizing patients based upon the diagnosis alone. We need to recall that the patient is an equal member of the Discharge Planning Team. Chapter 3 will discuss the patient's perspective in this process.

Table 2–1 Problem-Solving Methods

Area of conflict: The social work department believes a social worker should screen all patients initially, including skilled home care referrals.

Problem-Solving Type	*Approach*	*Solution*
Heuristic	Trial and Error	For the next 2 weeks, whoever sees the patient first has the initial contact and introduces the idea of discharge planning. Reevaluate if conflict occurs.
Experimentation	Scientific	On the third floor the social worker will make the initial contact. On the fourth floor the home care discharge planner will make the initial contact. Data will be collected and evaluated after 2 weeks.
Critique	Before/After	Evaluate pros and cons of above approach before and after implementation.
Gestalt	Whole Problem	It is possible that the respiratory therapist will make the initial contact if notified for home oxygen before involvement of other disciplines. To meet this approach, a hospital policy should state: "The initial assessment is completed by the professional staff who first interacts with the patient."
Metaphor	Free Association	Brainstorming session of all multidisciplinary team members is held to identify options.
Rational	Analytical Thinking	It is possible that any discipline could make the initial contact, but it is unrealistic to expect all disciplines to provide the same information. The discipline that provides the initial visit will document its responsibilities and actions. Other disciplines will refer to this documentation for their ongoing planning.

Discharge Planning for Home Health Care
Copyright © 1994, Aspen Publishers, Inc.

Exhibit 2–2 Principles of Problem Solving

- Communicate in a nonthreatening manner.
- Define the problem, and raise the level of awareness (see Exhibit 2–3).
- Listen actively. Avoid criticism and judgmental responses.
- Delegate minor problems.
- Focus on major problems.
- Don't solve when under stress.
- Relax and temporarily step back from highly emotional issues or an impasse.
- Use humor. Be playful and nonconforming.
- Realize that no one solution is 100 percent correct. Look for many right answers.
- Brainstorm alternative solutions and resulting short-term and long-term effects. Challenge the traditional methods and rules.
- Compromise. Negotiate for a win–win solution.
- Propose trial period solutions.
- Implement solutions quickly.
- Evaluate the effectiveness of the solution, and revise if necessary.
- Use communication barrier busters (see Exhibit 2–5).
- Nurture creative thinking.

Discharge Planning for Home Health Care
Copyright © 1994, Aspen Publishers, Inc.

Exhibit 2–3 Conflict Analysis Work Sheet

1. Describe the problem. ____________________

____

____

2. What are the sources of conflict? ____________________

____

____

3. Circle the areas of conflict.

Intrapersonal	Intragroup
Interpersonal	Intergroup

4. Circle the categories of conflict.

Facts   Methods   Goals   Values

5. Describe your role and position and the role and position of others affected. ____________________

____

____

____

____

6. List suggested solutions. ____________________

____

____

____

____

____

____

____

____

____

____

DISCHARGE PLANNING FOR HOME HEALTH CARE
Copyright © 1994, Aspen Publishers, Inc.

Exhibit 2–4 Barriers to Communication

- Verbiage
- Past experiences
- Values
- Past relationship with person with whom you are communicating
- Tone
- Nonverbal signals
- Feelings
- Temperament
- Cultural background
- Social status
- Data overload
- Selective perception
- Thinking ahead
- Credibility of the speaker
- Anticipating the rest of the message
- Distractions
- Perceptions

Diagram of Communication

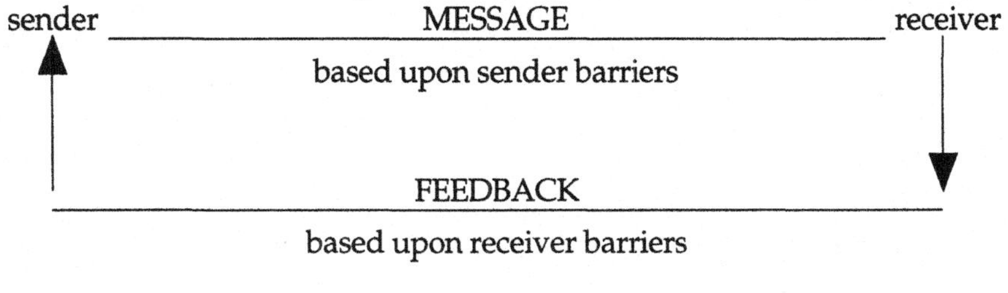

Barriers affect both written and oral communications. To minimize barriers, oral communication should also be provided in a written format. This can be followed by oral clarification of the subject matter. Using several formats of communication increase the percentage of successful communications.

DISCHARGE PLANNING FOR HOME HEALTH CARE
Copyright © 1994, Aspen Publishers, Inc.

Exhibit 2–5 Communication Barrier Busters

- Use silence to elicit feedback.
- Use open-ended questions.
- Listen for feelings, not just words.
- Restate what you think you heard (i.e., "Let me clarify. What you said was . . .").
- Avoid accusatory and aggressive comments (i.e., "You are looking for a scapegoat because you are lazy").
- Use the following techniques:
    - descriptive and assertive comments (i.e., "When you say the referrals are late again, I feel frustrated because I'm busy with the other responsibilities of my role and I feel as though I'm not meeting the expectations of my job")
    - negative assertion when admitting you are wrong (i.e., "You are right, it was inconsiderate to wait until 4:00 P.M. to call you with the information")
    - negative inquiry to elicit negative feedback (i.e., "Can you tell me how I can give you the referrals in a shorter time period on a consistent basis?")

DISCHARGE PLANNING FOR HOME HEALTH CARE
Copyright © 1994, Aspen Publishers, Inc.

Exhibit 2–6 Community Resource Questionnaire

Date____________________

Dear___________________________,

Can you please take a few minutes from you busy schedule to respond to our questions about our discharge planning services? You may add additional comments or suggestions on the back of this page if you desire. We have enclosed a stamped, self-addressed envelope for your convenience.

	Strongly Agree	**Agree**	**Unsure**	**Disagree**	**Strongly Disagree**
1. Referrals to your organization are timely.					
2. Referral information is complete.					
3. Information is useful.					
4. Care provided is care requested.					
5. Referrals to your organization are appropriate.					
6. Contact with our staff has been courteous and professional.					
7. You would recommend our organization to provide care for your patients.					
8. Feedback to you from our patients is positive.					

Suggestions to improve our services:____

Thank you for your assistance in evaluating our services!

Discharge Planning for Home Health Care
Copyright © 1994, Aspen Publishers, Inc.

◆ Appendix 2–A ◆

XYZ Hospital Discharge Plan

Policy: It is the policy of XYZ Hospital to provide high-risk patients with an individualized, comprehensive discharge plan that ensures continuity of care.

Definition: A multidisciplinary approach will be utilized to aid the transition of the patient's care from the hospital to an appropriate health care provider based upon the individual patient's medical, physical, social, and psychological needs. This process will begin no later than the patient's admission.

Goals:

1. Promote appropriate utilization of services.
2. Provide information to the patient necessary for informed decision making.
3. Provide a multidisciplinary approach by educating the patient and family and by formulating a comprehensive discharge plan.
4. Develop coordination with community resources to ensure continuity of care.
5. Provide assessment follow-up to all patients meeting screening criteria.
6. Evaluate effectiveness of discharge plans, and revise methodology if ineffective.

DISCHARGE PLANNING FOR HOME HEALTH CARE
Copyright © 1994, Aspen Publishers, Inc.

IDENTIFICATION OF DISCHARGE PLANNING TEAM MEMBERS

1. Patient
   - May include family
   - May include significant other
2. Physician
3. Nurse
4. Social Worker
5. Home Care Coordinator (Home Care Discharge Planner)
6. Physical Therapist
7. Occupational Therapist
8. Speech Therapist
9. Respiratory Therapist
10. Utilization Management Coordinator
11. Quality Improvement Coordinator
12. Dietitian
13. Pastoral Care Counselor
14. Finance Representative
15. Admissions Clerk

IDENTIFICATION OF COMMUNITY RESOURCES

1. Home Health Agencies
2. Area Agency on Aging (multiple programs)
3. Personal Care Homes
4. Skilled Nursing Facilities (SNFs)
5. Intermediate Care Facilities (ICFs)
6. Outpatient Therapy Services
7. Outpatient Ancillary Services
8. Office of Vocational Rehabilitation
9. Day care centers
10. Diagnosis specific community agencies
11. Meals on Wheels

REGULATIONS GOVERNING DISCHARGE PLANNING

1. Medicare
2. Department of Health, Education and Welfare
3. State assistance (Medicaid)
4. Joint Commission on Accreditation of Healthcare Organizations
5. Peer Review Organizations

SCREENING CRITERIA

All patients will be screened as early as possible to ascertain appropriateness of utilization and to begin discharge planning.

1. Any patient with any of the following diagnoses will be referred to the social service/home care department representative of the discharge planning team:
   _____cardiovascular accident
   _____fracture (multiple or major bone or joint)
   _____amputations
   _____myocardial infarctions
   _____recurrent angina
   _____second- or third-degree burns
   _____Alzheimer's or other mind-altering disease
   _____malignancies
   _____prosthesis (including ostomy)
   _____drainage tubes
   _____cardiac/respiratory arrest
   _____diabetes (uncontrolled or newly diagnosed)
   _____psychiatric problems
   _____extensive surgery
   _____congestive heart failure
   _____chronic obstructive pulmonary disease
   _____long-term ventilator support
2. Any patient with the following psychosocial problem will be referred immediately to social services:
   _____over 65 and living alone
   _____noncompliance with medical regime
   _____no known residence
   _____lack of support system
   _____inadequate financial support
   _____inadequate living arrangements
3. Patients in need of definite home care services will be referred immediately to the home care discharge planner/social worker as deemed appropriate:
   _____home IV therapy
   _____activities of daily living
   _____durable medical equipment
   _____nursing
   _____aide care
   _____therapy
   _____patient teaching
   _____social services
   _____current home care patients

4. Patients admitted from an extended care facility or ICF should be referred immediately to social services.
5. Patients readmitted within 30 days of hospital discharge should be referred immediately to social services/home care.
6. Patients admitted to pediatrics with any of the following should be referred immediately to social services:
   _____failure to thrive
   _____severe handicap
   _____repeated admissions
   _____questionable neglect/abuse
   _____poor home environment
   _____poor support systems
7. Newborns with the following problems should be referred immediately to social services or the home care discharge planner as appropriate:
   _____congenital anomalies
   _____requiring adoption/foster care placement
   _____severe handicaps
   _____high-risk mother
   _____patient who is HIV (Human Immunodeficiency Virus) positive
8. All requests from the patient and/or family should be referred immediately to appropriate team members.
9. All patients in the above high-risk categories accessing ambulatory care will be referred immediately to social services/home care discharge planner.

ROLES/RESPONSIBILITIES OF DISCHARGE PLANNING TEAM MEMBERS

1. Patient, family member, or significant other:
   - To read rights and responsibilities.
   - To cooperate with discharge planning team.
   - To assist with social/medical support needs after discharge.
2. Physician:
   - To admit and discharge the patient.
   - To order medical treatments.
   - To provide pertinent information about the patient's condition and psychosocial status.
   - To provide other members of the discharge planning team with 24-hour minimum notice of intent to discharge.
   - To write orders for follow-up care.
3. Nurse:
   - To complete the patient information profile on admission.
   - To assess the patient's medical, physical, and psychosocial needs and refer as indicated.
   - To initiate patient education.

- To act as a liaison between patient/family/physician/social worker and home care.
- To participate actively in discharge planning meetings.
- To complete an accurate discharge summary/instruction sheet.
- To contact the patient within 48 hours of discharge to ascertain status.

4. Social Worker:
   - To screen all admissions to identify high-risk patients.
   - To evaluate the patient within three calendar days, including complete psychosocial status.
   - To offer the patient a clear choice of providers (i.e., durable medical equipment companies).
   - To devise a plan and elicit patient/family support through the education and interview processes.
   - To provide the patient/family with information about available community resources.
   - To coordinate all SNF/ICF/personal care home placements.
   - To participate actively in weekly discharge planning meetings on all assigned units and family conferences when needed.
   - To document all discharge planning activities on the patient's medical record.
   - To communicate to all team members as deemed appropriate.
5. Home Care Coordinator:
   - To accept referrals from any source.
   - To review the patient record for appropriateness to home care.
   - To offer the patient a clear choice of home care providers while educating the patient about realistic plans/expectations.
   - To coordinate the patient's skilled and private duty home care plan.
   - To act as liaison between hospital and community home health providers.
   - To participate actively in weekly unit discharge planning meetings and family conferences when needed.
   - To communicate verbally and follow up with written signed referrals of all home care orders to the patient's provider of choice.
   - To document discharge planning activity on the patient's medical record.
   - To precertify insurance and verify coverage for home care.
   - To communicate to team members as deemed appropriate.
6. Physical Therapist: see below, Occupational Therapist
7. Occupational Therapist:
   - To assess patients for follow-up needs.
   - To provide home evaluations on an as needed basis.
   - To make recommendations to the physician and other appropriate discharge planning team members regarding need for follow-up care.
   - To educate the patient/family regarding follow-up.

- To participate actively in discharge planning meetings and family conferences when appropriate.
- To recommend patient equipment needs.
- To communicate to all discharge planning team members as deemed appropriate.
- To document all discharge planning activity on the patient's medical record.

8. Speech Therapist:
   - To assess all patients for follow-up needs.
   - To make recommendations to the physician and other discharge planning team members regarding need for follow-up care.
   - To educate the patient/family regarding need for follow-up care.
   - To participate actively in discharge planning meetings and family conferences when appropriate.
   - To document all discharge planning activity on the patient's medical record.
9. Respiratory Therapist:
   - To assess patients for potential follow-up needs.
   - To offer patients a clear choice of respiratory therapy providers.
   - To act as liaison among patient, hospital, and provider of choice.
   - To participate actively in discharge planning and family meetings when indicated.
   - To document all discharge planning activity on the patient's medical record.
10. Utilization Management Coordinator:
    - To perform precertification and ongoing review as mandated by public law.
    - To refer identified problems to appropriate members of the discharge planning team.
    - To evaluate the appropriate utilization of acute care and length of stay.
    - To monitor/assess documentation and recommend additional helpful but missing information.
    - To provide education to the patient, physician, and staff.
    - To participate actively in weekly unit discharge planning meetings.
11. Quality Improvement Coordinator:
    - To monitor effectiveness of the discharge planning process through the use of quality indicators.
    - To recommend changes in the process when the need arises.
12. Dietitian:
    - To assess patient status and potential follow-up needs.
    - To recommend follow-up to the physician.
    - To educate the patient, family, and staff.
    - To participate actively in patient conferences when indicated.
    - To document all discharge planning activity on the patient's medical record.
13. Pastoral Care Counselor:
    - To assess high-risk patients' spiritual needs.
    - To communicate needs to the discharge planning team as deemed appropriate.

14. Financial Representative:
    - To evaluate underinsured and uninsured patients for alternative financial resource planning when indicated.
    - To assist in decision making to offset larger loss when care can be provided safely in an alternative setting.
15. Admissions Clerk:
    - To complete pre-admission discharge planning work sheet.

MULTIDISCIPLINARY PATIENT DISCHARGE PLANNING CONFERENCES

1. A multidisciplinary patient discharge planning team conference will occur no less than weekly.
2. At minimum, the following team members will be present: nurse, social worker, home care coordinator, and utilization management coordinator.

DISCHARGE PLANNING TEAM MEETING FORMAT

1. The nurse will provide the patient's name, room number, diagnosis, and current status.
2. The nurse will offer any information about home setting, support systems, and possible needs.
3. The social worker will offer information from the psychosocial perspective.
4. Other team members will offer appropriate input.
5. A tentative plan will be established.
6. Discharge Planning Team members will follow up after the meeting.

◆ Chapter 3 ◆

The Patient's Perspective

The patient is a vital link in the discharge planning team. When patients find themselves faced with a change in body image as a result of their acute disease process, they sense fear of the unknown and an overwhelming loss of control. Consider the patient with a cerebrovascular accident (CVA). Last week, she had been creating a scenic environment as she landscaped around her large pond, which she views from the picture window of her restored farmhouse. After sharing a snack with her husband and watching television, she had retired for the night. This was a typical day. When she woke, she realized after a few moments that she was not at home. She could hear her husband speak yet found herself unable to respond. She couldn't see clearly because in the excitement everyone forgot that she wore both glasses and contacts, and her contacts had been left at home. She wanted to reach out and hold her husband, but she was unable to move. It would be days until she would understand that she had had a stroke and months until she could relay her story.

Melodramatic? Not at all. This is a true story, one that repeats itself daily in hospitals across the country with minor changes in the details. As health care providers, we must make an active attempt to consider the human side of illness. Our patients are not just "the CVA in room 119" or "the appendectomy in room 409." They are people, like you and me. They are accustomed to being in control of their bodies, their daily activities, and their lives. They have rights; legally and morally we have an obligation to promote the rights of our patients.

PATIENT RIGHTS

The American Hospital Association adopted the patient Bill of Rights in 1973. These are outlined in Exhibit 3–1. Item 10 addresses the patient's right to continuity of care. It is the patient's right to expect that the hospital has in place a mechanism to ensure this continuity of care and to provide complete information about continued health care needs after discharge. Of additional importance to the discharge planning process is the patient's right to confidentiality and the protection of his or her privacy. Most hospitals have general administrative policies stipulating access to records as authorized by the patient at the time of admission. Before information is shared with anyone not directly involved with the patient's care, it is best to obtain the patient's permission. Documentation of the discussion with the patient regarding release of information should be made on the medical record.

Release of information often becomes an issue when a third party payor provides case management and subsequently provides discharge planning. After discussing the role of the Discharge Planning Team and the role of the third party payor's case management, the hospital employee should document that the patient was informed that Jane Doe, the case manager for insurance company A, has requested information to plan posthospital care. The patient must be informed of the hospital's discharge planning team and available resources as well as the fact that Jane Doe represents the interests of insurance company A and not necessarily the interests of the hospital. The patient should indicate understanding and request that Jane Doe be provided with any needed information to plan for his or her postdischarge care.

The patient and his or her significant other need to know which professional is responsible for the various discharge planning tasks. They should be provided with:

- the full names and titles of those involved
- what discharge planning means (i.e., thinking about going home or leaving the hospital)
- the discharge planning team's problem-solving process
- the information that the physician determines the actual discharge date and is responsible for ordering posthospital discharge care
- the information that posthospital care is always available either through insurance, private pay, or third party payors (specifics must be discussed clearly to eliminate nonviable plans before discharge)
- information about the roles of the patient, the discharge planning team, and the family

SELF-ASSESSMENT

Either before hospitalization or at the time of admission, the patient should complete a self-assessment (Exhibit 3–2). This provides the discharge planning team with a baseline. Caution must be exercised because this is the patient's perspective; in many ways it may be the most reliable, and in other respects it may be unrealistic because of the emotional reaction to the

Exhibit 3–1 Patient Bill of Rights*

1. The patient has the right to considerate and respectful care.

2. The patient has the right to and is encouraged to obtain from physicians and other direct caregivers relevant, current, and understandable information concerning diagnosis, treatment, and prognosis.
   Except in emergencies when the patient lacks decision-making capacity and the need for treatment is urgent, the patient is entitled to the opportunity to discuss and request information related to the specific procedures and/or treatments, the risks involved, the possible length of recuperation, and the medically reasonable alternatives and their accompanying risks and benefits.
   Patients have the right to know the identity of physicians, nurses, and others involved in their care, as well as when those involved are students, residents, or other trainees. The patient also has the right to know the immediate and long-term financial implications of treatment choices, insofar as they are known.

3. The patient has the right to make decisions about the plan of care prior to and during the course of treatment and to refuse a recommended treatment or plan of care to the extent permitted by law and hospital policy and to be informed of the medical consequences of this action. In case of such refusal, the patient is entitled to other appropriate care and services that the hospital provides or transfer to another hospital. The hospital should notify patients of any policy that might affect patient choice within the institution.

4. The patient has the right to have an advance directive (such as a living will, health care proxy, or durable power of attorney for health care) concerning treatment or designating a surrogate decision maker with the expectation that the hospital will honor the intent of that directive to the extent permitted by law and hospital policy.
   Health care institutions must advise patients of their rights under state law and hospital policy to make informed medical choices, ask if the patient has an advance directive, and include that information in patient records. The patient has the right to timely information about hospital policy that may limit its ability to implement fully a legally valid advance directive.

5. The patient has the right to every consideration of privacy. Case discussion, consultation, examination, and treatment should be conducted so as to protect each patient's privacy.

6. The patient has the right to expect that all communications and records pertaining to his/her care will be treated as confidential by the hospital, except in cases such as suspected abuse and public health hazards when reporting is permitted or required by law. The patient has the right to expect that the hospital will emphasize the confidentiality of this information when it releases it to any other parties entitled to review information in these records.

7. The patient has the right to review the records pertaining to his/her medical care and to have the information explained or interpreted as necessary, except when restricted by law.

8. The patient has the right to expect that, within its capacity and policies, a hospital will make reasonable response to the request of a patient for appropriate and medically indicated care and

services. The hospital must provide evaluation, service, and/or referral as indicated by the urgency of the case. When medically appropriate and legally permissible, or when a patient has so requested, a patient may be transferred to another facility. The institution to which the patient is to be transferred must first have accepted the patient for transfer. The patient must also have the benefit of complete information and explanation concerning the need for, risks, benefits, and alternatives to such a transfer.

9. The patient has the right to ask and be informed of the existence of business relationships among the hospital, educational institutions, other health care providers, or payors that may influence the patient's treatment and care.

10. The patient has the right to consent to or decline to participate in proposed research studies or human experimentation affecting care and treatment or requiring direct patient involvement, and to have those studies fully explained prior to consent. A patient who declines to participate in research or experimentation is entitled to the most effective care that the hospital can otherwise provide.

11. The patient has the right to expect reasonable continuity of care when appropriate and to be informed by physicians and other caregivers of available and realistic patient care options when hospital care is no longer appropriate.

12. The patient has the right to be informed of hospital policies and practices that relate to patient care, treatment, and responsibilities. The patient has the right to be informed of available resources for resolving disputes, grievances, and conflicts, such as ethics committees, patient representatives, or other mechanisms available in the institution. The patient has the right to be informed of the hospital's charges for services and available payment methods.

*These rights can be exercised on the patient's behalf by a designated surrogate or proxy decision maker if the patient lacks decision-making capacity, is legally incompetent, or is a minor.

Notes: A Patient's Bill of Rights was first adopted by the American Hospital Association in 1973. This revision was approved by the AHA Board of Trustees on October 21, 1992.

Source: Reprinted with permission of the American Hospital Association, copyright © 1992.

Exhibit 3–2 Patient Self-Assessment

Completed: _____At time of admission

_____Pre-admission

1. I came to the hospital because:

2. At this time I feel_____as I normally do _____scared _____tense _____other (specify)

3. Before coming to the hospital, I needed help with:

_____bathing	_____meal preparation
_____shaving	_____toileting
_____mouth care	_____medical care (i.e., wound care)
_____cleaning	explain: ______________________
_____shopping	______________________
_____transportation	______________________
_____other (specify)	_____use of telephone

4. I am being helped by______________________at______________________.
name phone

5. I am using the following community agency support:

6. When I am discharged, I think I will:

_____need family/friend support only

_____need agency help

_____need a nursing facility

_____unsure at this time

Patient Name ______________________

Date Completed ______________________

PHYSICAL SELF-ASSESSMENT

Do you . . .	Yes	No	Comments
1. have pain?			
2. have trouble sleeping?			
3. have trouble walking?			
4. have trouble changing positions?			
5. have trouble seeing?			
6. wear glasses?			
7. wear contacts?			

DISCHARGE PLANNING FOR HOME HEALTH CARE
Copyright © 1994, Aspen Publishers, Inc.

Exhibit 3–2 continued

Do you . . .	Yes	No	Comments
8. have trouble hearing?			
9. wear a hearing aid?			
10. wear dentures?			
partial?			
full?			
11. have trouble chewing?			
12. have trouble swallowing?			
13. have an appetite?			
14. have other medical problems in addition to current reason for hospitalization?			
15. smoke?			
16. do breast self-exams? (if female)			
17. do testicular exams? (if male)			
Did you . . .			
1. have a Pap smear in the past year?			
2. have a rectal exam in the past year?			
Are you . . .			
1. on a special diet?			
2. on fluid precautions?			
Do you . . .			
1. have food preferences?			
2. drink caffeine?			
3. have food allergies or sensitivities?			
4. drink alcohol beverages?			
5. urinate more than 6 times a day?			
6. get up at night to urinate?			
7. leak urine?			
8. have daily bowel movements?			
9. need routine laxatives or enemas?			
10. have medication allergies or sensitivities?			
11. have other allergies or sensitivities?			
12. take any medication not prescribed by a physician? (specify below)			

DISCHARGE PLANNING FOR HOME HEALTH CARE
Copyright © 1994, Aspen Publishers, Inc.

Exhibit 3–2 continued

Do you . . .	Yes	No	Comments
13. take medication prescribed by a physician? (specify below)			

Medication	*Dose*	*Frequency*	*Last Dose*

SOCIAL SELF-ASSESSMENT

1. Currently I live with _____spouse _____other relative _____parent(s) _____friend _____child(ren) _____alone _____other (specify)
2. I live in a(n): _____private home on: _____1 floor _____apartment _____2 floors or more _____boarding home _____skilled nursing home
3. Next of kin, address and phone: ______________________________

____

Relationship: ______________________________

PSYCHOLOGICAL SELF-ASSESSMENT

Do you . . .	Yes	No	Comments
1. become upset often?			
2. become irritable often?			
3. have emotional problems that you are aware of?			
4. have concerns about home because you are in the hospital?			
5. have personal concerns you want to discuss?			
6. have other problems? (specify)			

Discharge Planning for Home Health Care
Copyright © 1994, Aspen Publishers, Inc.

Exhibit 3–2 continued

MISCELLANEOUS SELF-ASSESSMENT

1. My religion is ______________________

Do you . . .	Yes	No	Comments
1. have special religious requests?			
2. have an organ donor card?			
3. have a living will?			
4. want information about your illness? your medications? how to stop smoking? how to control your weight? living wills? advance directives? organ donations? stress management?			
5. have a durable medical power of attorney appointed? If yes, specify: Name ______ Address ______ ______ Telephone ______ Relationship ______			
6. want to talk to a member of the discharge planning team? (specify)			

Directions: 1 copy for patient record

DISCHARGE PLANNING FOR HOME HEALTH CARE
Copyright © 1994, Aspen Publishers, Inc.

stress from the hospitalization. It is recommended that the patient's primary nurse be responsible for overseeing the completion of this assessment in conjunction with his or her initial nursing assessment. This helps develop rapport with the patient. The nurse can address any concerns or unclear answers during the initial interview process.

FAMILY DYNAMICS

Although a supportive family actively participates in the team's planning efforts, we need to recognize that family interactions are as consistent during illness as they are during wellness. Often there is an underlying history among family members that is not reported or is inaccurately reported to the planning team. At times, these "skeletons" contribute to the hesitation on the part of the family and unrealistic expectations of the patient. Each patient and family brings histories and beliefs with them that form their actions and reactions. All planning team members must be empathetic with regard to the dynamics of the family.

LEVELS OF CARE

Many times the patient's perspective does not correlate with today's level of health care. There are utilization management activities in health care today with the goal of appropriate utilization of facilities to promote the cost-effective delivery of care. The four levels or categories of care for the patient are:

Level of Care	*Facility*	*Criteria*
Acute*	Hospital	New onset of illness Acute exacerbation of chronic illness Major injury Requires evaluation and new treatment
Skilled*	Rehabilitation facility Skilled nursing facility Home care Hospice	Seriousness of acute nature is over Ongoing need for supportive services
Intermediate*	Intermediate care facility Home care Hospice	Rehabilitation is complete Patient requires some support but has achieved greater independence With the exception of hospice, expect that patient will improve
Custodial†	Personal care facility Home care	Patient requires help with activities of daily living Chronic stable condition Not expected that patient will improve

*Medicare/Medical assistance funding available within guidelines.
†Medical assistance funding available within guidelines.

PERCEPTIONS OF ILLNESS AND CARE

Frequently the patient and family have misconceptions regarding the health care system and the financing of care within the broad spectrum of health care settings. Some of this stems from the government's presentation of Medicare at its inception. Older patients vividly recall being told that Medicare would cover all their health needs once they reached 65.

Those currently approaching that age now have expectations that a third party will cover whatever is needed.

Family conferences (including the patient unless contraindicated) allow the discharge planning team to discuss the following:

- disease process
- recovery (actual and expected)
- potential needs/levels of care needed
- available options
- roles and expectations of patient, family, and health care providers within alternative settings
- financial considerations of alternative settings
- safety issues of alternative settings if applicable

As health care providers, we are responsible for educating the public about issues concerning illness in the health care arena of today. Public support or concern should be expressed to Congress by relaying specific examples of health care needs and situations as they occur. An example of follow-up communication to families regarding proactive legislative actions is given in Exhibit 3–3. Legislative changes result not only from contacts by special interest groups but also from individuals communicating their specific concerns. Their contact probably cannot affect their current situation but may affect necessary changes in the future.

Because each individual is unique, Exhibit 3–4 outlines the patient's (and family's) perceptions of illness and health care. Table 3–1 describes some of the theories that explain a patient's behavior and access to care. It is important to consider the learning process in patient and family interactions (Exhibit 3–5).

Exhibit 3–3 Sample Follow-Up Communication Regarding Proactive Legislation

Mr. John Q. Public
100 East New Street
Anytown, USA 12345–6789

Dear Mr. Public,

As a follow up to our phone conversation on October 25, 1991, I want to restate my agreement with you that there are many people with chronic debilitating needs in their homes today requiring custodial care. I am pleased that our agency was able to provide private duty services for your mother on a private pay basis. Often, health care consumers realize the lack of funding at a time of need when personal situations arise. Agency A is a member of Pennsylvania Association of Home Health Agencies and also the National Association of Home Care. All home care providers actively support upcoming long-term care legislation that would help thousands of Americans in situations similar to your mother's. I am in hopes that you will write to your senators in support of:

Senate Bill 375

- Will set minimum standards for long-term care insurance providers
- Introduced by the State Banking and Insurance Committee

Senate Bill 377

- Mandates the giving of the option to purchase home care in all health insurance policies
- Introduced by the Senate Banking and Insurance Committee

A list of Pennsylvania legislators and their addresses has been attached. Thank you for your understanding of this troubling area in today's health care arena.

Sincerely,

Jane Smith, Administrative Director

Discharge Planning for Home Health Care
Copyright © 1994, Aspen Publishers, Inc.

Exhibit 3–4 Patient/Family Perception of Illness

Factors affecting perceptions of illness, health care utilization, and follow-up assistance include:

- age
- sex
- ethnic background
- culture
- beliefs/attitudes
- education level
- social class
- past experiences
- emotional reaction
- cost of treatment
  1. reimbursement
     —insurance
     —third party
     —self-pay
  2. financial status
- availability of care
  1. reputation
  2. hours
  3. location
- effect of illness
  1. alteration in activities of daily living
  2. level of pain
  3. perceived threat
- knowledge of the symptoms
  1. advice from others
  2. mass media
  3. articles

DISCHARGE PLANNING FOR HOME HEALTH CARE
Copyright © 1994, Aspen Publishers, Inc.

Table 3–1 Theories of Patient Behavior

Theorist	*Theory Synopsis*
Kosa and Robertson	Focus is the psychological need to reduce anxiety through: • values application to the effects of the illness on daily activities • anxiety related to the patient's perception • application of the patient's medical knowledge • interventions to alleviate anxiety
Suchman	Focus is the sociological perspective through recognition that: • the patient has a symptom • the patient assumes the sick role • the patient seeks medical care • the patient assumes the dependent patient role • the patient recovers
Mechanic	Focus is broad with a variety of factors (social and psychological): • awareness of abnormal signs and symptoms • degree of seriousness is assigned to the symptoms • frequency of signs/symptoms • extent of disruption in daily routine • individual's level of tolerance to signs/symptoms • a focus on the available information and the patient's understanding of the disease • an understanding of the basic needs that create denial • recognition of competition between needs and response to illness • understanding of the variations in interpretation of signs/symptoms • knowledge of the availability and ease of access to health care

Discharge Planning for Home Health Care
Copyright © 1994, Aspen Publishers, Inc.

Exhibit 3–5 The Learning Process

1. **The environment should be:**
   - free of distraction (e.g., no television)
   - appropriate for what is being taught (e.g., the occupational therapist cannot teach meal preparation in the patient's hospital room)

2. **The teacher should:**
   - promote a relaxed atmosphere
   - determine the learner's current knowledge base
   - attempt to teach when the learner is least tired
   - convey a message consistent with that of other team members
   - be flexible and open to interruptions for questions
   - clarify learning objectives
   - develop a trusting relationship
   - listen actively to concerns of the learner
   - provide enough time to cover the topic (e.g., don't look rushed)
   - provide written instructions to reinforce verbal instructions
   - provide examples when appropriate
   - use teaching props available
   - introduce material in small portions to allow for absorption and retention
   - elicit feedback frequently

3. **The learner should:**
   - listen attentively
   - ask for clarification if unsure
   - offer information about self (including learning habits)
   - read written material
   - list questions in the absence of the teacher for future clarification
   - discuss fears and concerns with the teacher

The teacher–learner relationship is vital to learning.

DISCHARGE PLANNING FOR HOME HEALTH CARE
Copyright © 1994, Aspen Publishers, Inc.

◆ Chapter 4 ◆

The Home Care Coordination Perspective

WHY HAVE A HOME CARE COORDINATOR POSITION?

For the patient returning to the home environment, it is essential that the discharge plan be thoroughly coordinated and allowed to evolve throughout the hospital stay. Traditionally, the hospital social worker was responsible for the coordination of all posthospital plans. The volumes of referrals often necessitated that the referral was made on the day of patient discharge. This unavoidable delay in involving the home care agency resulted at best in a workable plan and at worst in an unsafe, incomplete, and unrealistic plan for both patient and provider. When glitches are recognized too late for correction, discharge planning is ineffective and results in frustrations and apprehensions for the patient, his or her caregivers, and the agency.

Who is the most qualified person to plan for the patient's return home? Logically, this person should be knowledgeable in home care admission criteria, regulations, reimbursement criteria, available programs, in-home safety issues, and the roles of the family and agency personnel. This role can most appropriately be carried out by an experienced home care nurse. The title for this person could be home care coordinator, home care liaison, home care discharge planner, or any other title that fits well with the overall organizational chart. For our purposes, we will call this individual the Home Care Coordinator. Acting as a liaison between the patient and his or her current and future caregivers, the Home Care Coordinator possesses the expertise to ensure a viable and safe plan.

ORGANIZATIONAL PLACEMENT

A major obstacle with incorporation of the Home Care Coordinator role into the Discharge Planning Team results from the turf issues that often arise with the social worker. The Task Force helps determine organizational placement of the Home Care Coordinator, which conveys the value placed upon the role, molds internal and external perceptions of the role, determines the amount of autonomy of the role, and implies the loyalties of the role (i.e., to the hospital or home care department).

Seven organizational options, each with its pros and cons regarding the placement of the Home Care Coordinator, are given in Figures 4–1 to 4–7. In the first two options the position is a part of the Social Services department. Note that option 1 places the Home Care Coordinator as an equal to the social worker, thus implying equal value, whereas option 2 devalues the position by making it a subordinate to the social worker. Options 3 and 4 place the position within the Home Care department at different levels. The newly organized department would probably utilize option 3 until an increase in the referral base required an intake supervisor for hospital home care coordination and outside referral base coordination. Option 5 places the position as a part of administration. This would be most likely to occur in a small hospital. Option 6 places the Home Care Coordinator under an overall Quality Assessment department which encompasses the traditional departments of Utilization Management, Social Services, Infection Surveillance, and Risk Management. In this option our Home Care Coordinator would function under the Discharge Planning Coordinator/Supervisor. Option 7 recognizes the interdependence of discharge coordination with Utilization Management and places the Home Care Coordinator as an equal to all review and planning personnel. Your hospital may have institution-specific pros and cons to add to the developed lists that follow.

ROLES AND RESPONSIBILITIES

It is imperative for the Home Care Coordinator role to function independently because dependence upon others for direction and patient access can affect timeliness and effectiveness of discharge planning. Delayed intervention negatively affects effective planning and coordination and is often the sole reason for a plan that disintegrates as the patient is wheeled out the door. The patient and his or her family or significant others need time physically and mentally to prepare themselves for discharge. In essence, their acceptance of the plan is instrumental to its effectiveness, and only through active, ongoing participation will there be acceptance of the plan.

The coordinator will incorporate payor source criteria into the patient's discharge plan. Medicare and some state medical assistance programs require the patient to be homebound; there are various interpretations of this criterion. Government-funded programs and other third party payors require documentation of a medical need for skilled care with a developed plan of care, including goals. Although the plan cannot be complete until the patient is

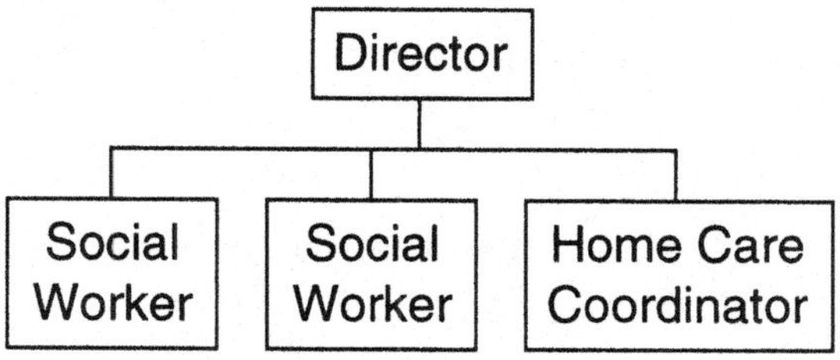

Pros	*Cons*
1. Perceived by staff as important to discharge planning	1. Alliance is to Social Services Department, thus decreasing recognition of home health needs
2. Independent role	2. Delay in updates regarding regulatory changes
3. All discharge planning personnel are within the same department	3. Inservices not geared toward home care coordination needs
4. Role in discharge planning evident to outside providers	

Figure 4–1 Organizational Option 1: Social Services Department.

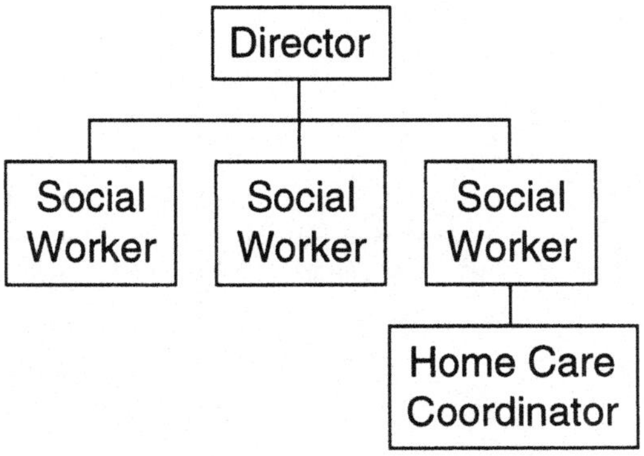

Pros	*Cons*
1. All discharge planning personnel are within the same department	1. Dependent role
2. Role in discharge planning evident to outside provider	2. Alliance is to Social Services department, thus decreasing recognition of home health needs
	3. Potential for devaluation of position by hospital staff
	4. Delay in updates regarding regulatory changes
	5. Inservices not geared to home care coordination

Figure 4–2 Organizational Option 2: Social Services Department.

Copyright © 1994, Aspen Publishers, Inc.

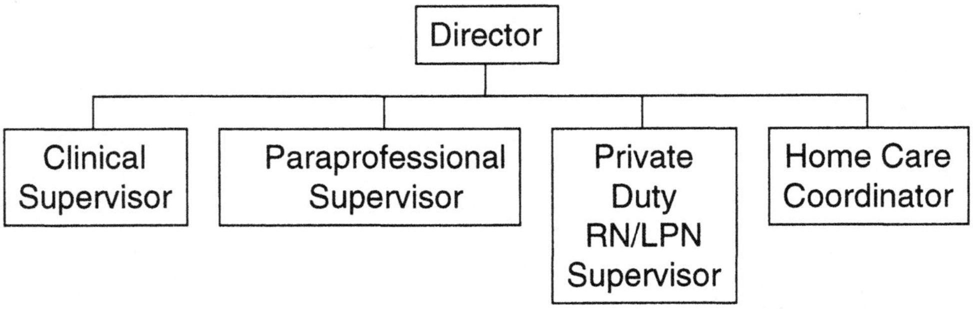

Pros

1. Alliance is to home care
2. Perceived as an independent hospital role
3. Timely receipt of updates regarding home care regulations
4. Inservices/continuing education directed toward home health arena

Cons

1. Role confusion among hospital staff
2. Potential for role dependency
3. Potential for outside agencies to question patient freedom of choice

Figure 4–3 Organizational Option 3: Home Care Department.

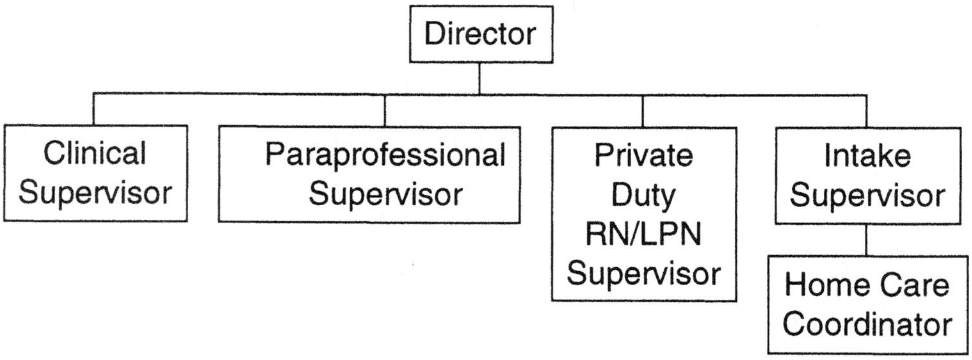

Pros

1. Alliance is to home care
2. Perceived as an independent hospital role
3. Timely receipt of updates of regulatory changes
4. Inservices/continuing education directed toward home health arena

Cons

1. Role confusion among hospital staff
2. Potential for role dependency
3. Potential for outside agencies to question patient freedom of choice

Figure 4–4 Organizational Option 4: Home Care Department.

DISCHARGE PLANNING FOR HOME HEALTH CARE
Copyright © 1994, Aspen Publishers, Inc.

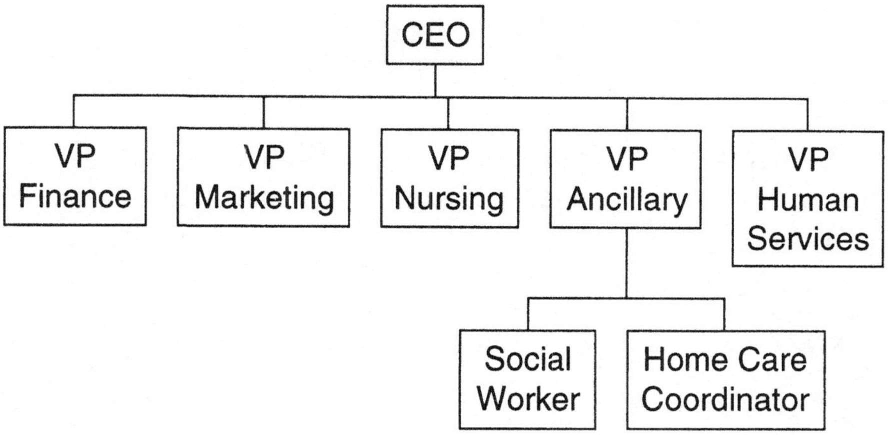

Pros	*Cons*
1. Perceived by hospital staff as valuable to discharge planning 2. Alliance is to patient and hospital 3. Independent role 4. Role in discharge planning is evident to outside providers	1. Delay in updates regarding regulatory changes 2. Importance of home care coordinator can be lost in administrative priorities 3. Inservices/continuing education not geared to home health coordination needs

Figure 4–5 Organizational Option 5: Administration.

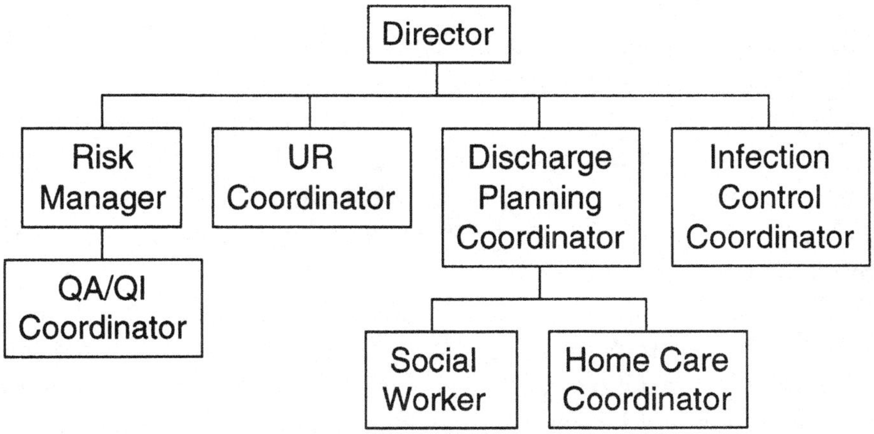

Pros	*Cons*
1. All discharge planning personnel are within the same department 2. Perceived by hospital staff as valuable to discharge planning 3. Independent role 4. Role in discharge planning evident to outside providers 5. Alliance is to patient and hospital	1. Delay in updates regarding regulatory changes 2. Inservices/continuing education not geared toward home health coordination

Figure 4–6 Organizational Option 6: Quality Assessment Department.

DISCHARGE PLANNING FOR HOME HEALTH CARE
Copyright © 1994, Aspen Publishers, Inc.

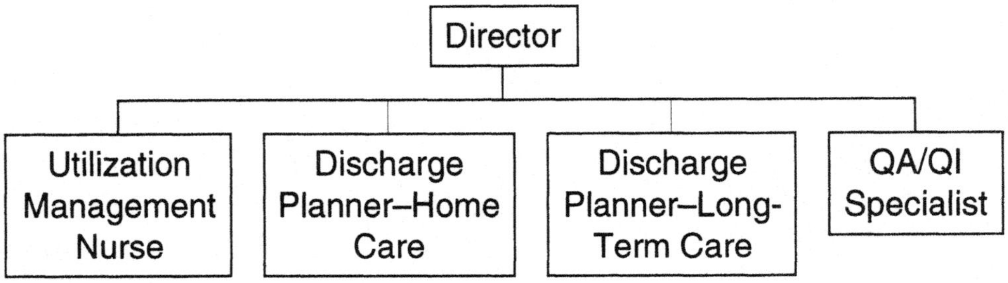

Pros	*Cons*
1. All discharge planning personnel are within the same department 2. Perceived by hospital staff as valuable to discharge planning 3. Independent role 4. Role in discharge planning evident to outside providers 5. Alliance is to patient and hospital	1. Delay in updates regarding regulatory changes 2. Inservices/continuing education not geared toward home health coordination

Figure 4–7 Organizational Option 7: Utilization Management Department.

assessed in the home care environment, the Home Care Coordinator is solely responsible for its initial inception. Benefit negotiations with insurance companies on an individual basis are part of this role. The outcome is provision of cost-effective care in the setting most conducive to the patient's situation. For this to be prosperous for all, the insurance company representative must be empowered with the ability to make independent decisions. Regardless of the payment source, the Home Care Coordinator's knowledge of the reimbursement criteria is essential for viable home care referrals.

While utilizing his or her knowledge, the independently functioning home care coordinator has the authority to pursue optimal dispositions. Because it is sometimes too easy to decide in 60 seconds or less what we, as health care practitioners, believe is in the best interest of our patients, we must not lose sight of the fact that our patients need to make their own decisions. As an example, let's look at Mr. Jones, an 80-year-old patient with chronic obstructive pulmonary disease who was ventilator dependent for 2 weeks secondary to respiratory failure. The Home Care Coordinator became aware of his situation from weekly discharge planning meetings, and staff expectations were that he would require temporary placement in a skilled nursing facility to build his strength. Mrs. Jones, his 90-pound frail-looking wife, had different expectations. Specifically, she planned to take her husband home and care for him as she had always promised.

The astute Home Care Coordinator spent much time with Mr. and Mrs. Jones to impress upon them what would be necessary and required of them for a home recovery. Together they decided to have a 24-hour trial phase in the hospital. The Home Care Coordinator arranged for a staff nurse to have a light assignment to allow for the necessary time to provide complete step-by-step patient care instructions to Mrs. Jones. Mrs. Jones came to the realization that she not only had an enormous amount of love for her husband but also that she was physically capable of caring for him at home with moderate assistance. She couldn't afford private duty care, but there were relatives and friends available to assist in the provision of the 24-hour care needed initially. A short-term trial home care placement was arranged.

The time the Home Care Coordinator spent with this couple was invaluable because the hospital was able to prevent an unsafe, nonworkable discharge plan. The rapport established with the Home Care Coordinator was the driving force behind the patient's acceptance of a trial home care discharge plan. The Home Care Coordinator also arranged for contact with a social worker who would contact the patient should this trial discharge plan be deemed unsafe at a later time.

As regulations change, the Home Care Coordinator offers alternative options to institutionalization because he or she immediately incorporates new regulations into planning. In summary, allowing the role of the Home Care Coordinator to function independently results in timely, comprehensive referrals with well-informed patients and caregivers.

In tailoring the individual plan, the Home Care Coordinator has a responsibility to the hospital, the patient, and the home care agency. As stated in Chapter 1, the hospital is mandated to provide discharge planning and will benefit from a reputation of quality and caring as the news of happy customers spreads. The needs of the hospital and the patient have been discussed in previous chapters. Now let's focus on the needs of the home care agency and how the Home Care Coordinator helps meet these needs.

Home care agencies need a comprehensive and accurate written referral that incorporates the patient's health care needs with pertinent psychosocial and financial data. The timely delivery of durable medical equipment and needed supplies to the patient's home must be coordinated. The agency wants to feel confident that teaching was started while the patient was in the hospital. There is nothing more frustrating for the patient and embarrassing for the hospital than the patient who goes home with an indwelling catheter and is unable to empty the bag. Often the Home Care Coordinator's gentle reminder to the busy hospital staff is the impetus needed for teaching to occur. The patient and agency expect that enough information was provided to delineate the roles and expectations of all caregivers involved to cultivate a viable plan.

The Home Care Coordinator has an alliance to the home care agency and is responsible and accountable for the easy transition from acute care to home care. This is the only role within the hospital system with this as its primary focus. A complete job description is included for reference in Appendix 4–A. Given the specificity of the tasks, it is easy to recognize that these time-consuming functions cannot be included in the role of the increasingly busy social worker, although collaboration with the social worker is an important part of the Home Care Coordinator's job.

CANDIDATE SELECTION

Selection of the right candidate for the home care coordinator position is of paramount importance to the candidate's acceptance of the role. The interview process offers a good time to weed out those lacking necessary qualifications. The interview question guide provided in Exhibit 4–1 will assist during the interview and will help determine the candidate's adaptability to the position. Professionalism is an important aspect of this position, so that attire and personality must be considered in selecting the right applicant to coordinate the health care needs of the patients.

Ideally, the selected candidate will have a minimum of 2 years of experience in the home care field, be motivated and organized, enjoy educating others about home care, have good interpersonal and marketing skills to collaborate with the members of the discharge planning team on both a professional and an informal level, and have specific career and personal goals. Reference checks will help separate those who interview well from those who function well.

Once hired, the Home Care Coordinator must become knowledgeable about all hospital departmental programs and the various local community resources. An awareness of the roles within the discharge planning team will help in the formulation of appropriate discharge plans.

ANTITRUST ISSUES

When hospital services include hospital-based home care, antitrust issues become a concern. To avoid legal ramifications, the hospital is required to offer a choice of home care providers. The Home Care Coordinator is the most appropriate position to offer the choice based upon his or her knowledge of home care and role as liaison with all providers. The spirit of the law is to ensure that all patients are provided with a choice of provider agencies. The method is left to the discretion of the hospital. Some hospitals' reactions to the fear of antitrust lawsuits have been ultraconservative, so that those patients without a preference are referred systematically among alternative providers. Some hospitals choose to provide a written list of all potential providers, whereas others offer only a verbal choice. The Home Care Coordinator must be certain to state that the hospital program is a department of the hospital. He or she can also feel confident and ethical in referring those without a stated preference to the hospital's department. The offering of a choice and the patient's response must be documented as part of the patient record.

PAST RELATIONSHIPS WITH HOME CARE PROVIDERS

Some patients may have a past relationship with a particular provider, which should be addressed in hospital policies. To promote positive community relationships, the hospital may want to consider the reasonable expectations of all outside providers. For instance, if the

Exhibit 4–1 Interviewer Question Guide

1. What is your health care background? Any specific to home health? Any coordination experience?
2. How would you describe your typical day's work? Do you:
   - organize the day the night before?
   - take things as they come?
   - wait for projects to come your way?
   - other (explain)
3. If your work hits a lull, what do you do?
   - Take a well-deserved coffee break.
   - Go to the next office and chat with the nurses.
   - Look for a new project.
   - Spend quiet time thinking about day-to-day operations and how to change.
4. Have you had the opportunity to speak before any groups? If so:
   - size?
   - type?
   - topic?
   - how did you feel?
5. What ways do you think we can market this position to the hospital? What problems do you foresee?
6. What expansion areas do you foresee for home care?
7. What has been your most difficult professional experience? How did you handle it?
8. Describe your actions when you have been unsure of the procedure to follow.
9. What are your personal goals?
10. What are your professional/career goals?
11. Describe yourself.

Copyright © 1994, Aspen Publishers, Inc.

patient is a current patient of a particular agency or has been discharged in the past 10 days, the hospital representative will initially talk with the patient to determine whether a satisfactory relationship existed and, if agreeable, refer posthospital care back to that provider. The hospital needs to be consistent in the application of its policy. The current home care provider needs to contact the home care coordinator as soon as possible with specific information when a patient is hospitalized. Exhibit 4–2 is an example of a written report that the provider can mail or fax to the Home Care Coordinator. It will be retained in the department office files.

COORDINATION TOOLS

At the end of this chapter are helpful working tools for the Home Care Coordinator to use. Carbonless copies of these forms are helpful for ease of communication.

1. Kardex flag (Exhibit 4–3): Placed on the patient Kardex on the nursing unit to alert staff of the potential for home care or a specific plan; includes information that is needed at the time of discharge for the referral to be complete; discard after discharge occurs
2. Coordination work sheet (Exhibit 4–4): Used to retrieve hospital information to enhance continuity of care from hospital to home; forward to the home care provider at time of discharge
3. Home care referral (Exhibit 4–5): Contains necessary intake information for the home care agency; forward original to the home care provider at time of discharge; one copy remains on the chart, one copy remains with the Home Care Coordinator files
4. Insurance work sheet (Exhibit 4–6): Provides the agency with necessary billing information; after a verbal explanation, the patient signs the form and receives a copy for his or her records; the original is forwarded to the home care provider
5. Interdepartmental communication sheet (Exhibit 4–7): Used to obtain information from specific members of the discharge planning team to obtain their expertise and input for incorporation into the discharge plan; discard after discharge
6. Patient information handout (Exhibit 4–8): Written information pertaining to home care and reimbursement sources that is given to the patient at the time of referral
7. Postdischarge communication (Exhibit 4–9): Given to the home care provider to elicit feedback about the patient's response to the home setting and information regarding deficiencies in discharge planning; may be used as part of the quality improvement plan
8. Monthly statistical report (Exhibit 4–10): Used to report statistical information to the department head and administration; retained on file in the department office

Exhibit 4–2 Home Health Agency Active Patient Status Checklist

Patient Name:____

Address: ____

____

____

____

Admitted to: ____

Currently receiving the following skilled service:

_____Nursing

_____Therapy (physical, occupational, speech)

_____Social services

_____Aide

_____Other (specify) ______________________________

____

____

____

____

Family dynamics:____

____

____

____

Please address the following concerns: ______________________________

____

____

Please contact____________________at________________for future home care needs.
Liaison Person Phone

Discharge Planning for Home Health Care
Copyright © 1994, Aspen Publishers, Inc.

Exhibit 4–3 Kardex Flag (Larger than Actual Size)

____

Patient Name

_____Prior to hospitalization this patient received home care from ____________________(agency).

_____The potential exists for this patient to need home care after discharge.

_____The home care referral is on the record. Please ask the physician to sign.

_____The home care referral has been signed. A copy is on the patient record for your convenience.

The patient will receive services from______________________________(agency)

at_______________(phone). PLEASE ADD THIS INFORMATION TO THE DISCHARGE INSTRUCTION SHEET.

AT THE TIME OF DISCHARGE, PLEASE:

_____Ask the physician for the following orders: ______________________________

____

____

____

_____Send the following supplies:______________________________

____

____

____

NOTIFY THE____________________DEPARTMENT AT EXTENSION #__________OR THE HOME CARE COORDINATOR (BEEPER #)__________________AT THE TIME OF DISCHARGE.

THANK YOU FOR YOUR ASSISTANCE IN THE DISCHARGE PROCESS!

____

Home Care Coordinator

Kardex Use—Discard after discharge

DISCHARGE PLANNING FOR HOME HEALTH CARE
Copyright © 1994, Aspen Publishers, Inc.

Exhibit 4–4 Coordination Work Sheet

Patient Name ______________________________ Room ______________

Directions to home ____

____

____

____

____

Lab Values	X-ray/Special Study Results

History (including dates of onset/surgery):

Synopsis of hospitalization:

Physician expectations of home care:

Patient/family dynamics:

Status of patient instruction:

Forward to home care provider at time of referral.

Discharge Planning for Home Health Care
Copyright © 1994, Aspen Publishers, Inc.

Exhibit 4–5 Home Care Referral

TBA ______________________________

Patient Name ______________________________

Address ______________________________

____

Phone ______________________________

1 Dx ______________________________

2 Dx ______________________________

____

Surgery ______________________________

____

Hospital Admin__________ D/C__________

Physician ______________________________

Allergies ______________________________

Equipment/supplies ______________________________

SKILLED NURSING

_____V/S _____Med teaching

_____Other (explain) ______________________________

____

____

Labs: ______________________________

Meds: ______________________________

____

____

____

IV care

_____Peripheral _____Central

_____Pump _____SASH

_____Instruct pt/significant other

Change: angio ______________________________

dressing ______________________________

AIDE

_____Personal care

_____Other

____

Physician signature Date

Please hold referral for pick-up.

Home care coordinator beeper # ______________________________

Voice mail # ______________________________

E-Mail # ______________________________

Referral Date ______________________________

Date of Birth ______________________________

Insurance ______________________________

____

____

SS # ______________________________

Mental status ______________________________

Prognosis ______________________________

Pt. aware? Yes No

Functional limitations

____

____

Diet ______________________________

Supplier ______________________________

Circle if given to pt:

Bill of rights

Agency phone #

Brochure Plan of care

Insurance criteria/benefits

PHYSICAL THERAPY

_____Assessment

_____Exercise program

_____Gait instruction

_____ROM _____Other

OCCUPATIONAL THERAPY

_____Assessment

_____Muscle reeducation

_____ADLs _____Other

SPEECH THERAPY

_____Assessment

_____Language

_____Other ______________________________

MSS ______________________________

____

PRIVATE DUTY

Level of care ______________________________

Hours ______________________________

Orders ______________________________

____

Original—Forward to home care provider

Copies: HCC/patient record

DISCHARGE PLANNING FOR HOME HEALTH CARE
Copyright © 1994, Aspen Publishers, Inc.

Exhibit 4–6 Insurance Work Sheet

Patient Name ____________________ SS# ____________________ Requested services
OT ST MSS AIDE
PD HMK CMP SN PT

Policyholder's name ____________________
SS# ____________________
Insurance company name ____________________
Address ____________________
Policy number ____________________
Employer ____________________
Address ____________________
Insurance contact ____________________
Phone ____________________

Requested supplies ____________________
____
Billing address ____________________
____
Terms of coverage ____________________
____
____
Deductible ____________________ Met/not met
Send with bill ____________________

THIS ACKNOWLEDGES THAT I RECEIVED A COPY OF THIS FORM WITH A VERBAL EXPLANATION

____
Patient Signature

Follow-up date due	Report of current status	Contact person	By:	Approved for:

Original—home care provider   Copy—Patient

Discharge Planning for Home Health Care
Copyright © 1994, Aspen Publishers, Inc.

Exhibit 4–7 Interdepartmental Communication Sheet

To: ______________________________ Department

In reviewing ______________________________ 's record, I have identified a potential need
(patient)

for follow-up home care. Can you please forward your proposed plan for PT, OT, ST, MSS, RT, Dietary, and Stomal Therapy in the space provided. If you can't write your plan and goals by

____________________, please page me on pager # ____________________.
(date)

Thank you for your assistance in developing an appropriate and comprehensive discharge plan.

____

____

____

____

____

____

____

____

____
Home Care Coordinator

Discard after discharge

DISCHARGE PLANNING FOR HOME HEALTH CARE
Copyright © 1994, Aspen Publishers, Inc.

Exhibit 4–8 Patient Information Handout

To our Valued Patient:

____________________________________ Hospital provides discharge planning for all patients in the hope that we can ensure continuity of your care and a speedy recovery. Through this planning process, we have identified some potential health care needs that we have discussed with you. We will be in contact with your physician to determine his or her agreement with our plans at this point. If he or she agrees that you will benefit from some home health follow-up, I will discuss your specific plan of care in more detail with you.

Most insurance companies pay a major portion of your home care bill, but be assured that we will do a complete investigation and give you a copy of our findings before you leave the hospital. Medicare and medical assistance patients need to be homebound, which is interpreted to mean that because of a physical condition you are unable to leave your home without great effort or assistance. As long as you require what these payors consider covered skilled care and remain homebound, your visits are paid in full.

Attached you will find a copy of the patient Rights and Responsibilities for your review. We can discuss any questions you may have about these rights and responsibilities, your payment source, home care plan, or any other concerns you may have during our next meeting. Should your family have questions for me, I can be reached at ____________________________.
(phone)

Sincerely,

____
Home Care Coordinator

Discharge Planning for Home Health Care
Copyright © 1994, Aspen Publishers, Inc.

Exhibit 4–9 Postdischarge Communication

____
Date

Dear __________________________,

We admitted __________________ to our agency for home care services on __________________. We found the discharge planning to be: _____complete

_____incomplete (specify)

____

____

____

Please relay to the staff on unit _________ that the patient is: _____doing well

_____having some difficulties (specify)

____

____

____

____

____

Sincerely,

Case Manager

________________________Agency

Return to Hospital A Home Care Coordinator

DISCHARGE PLANNING FOR HOME HEALTH CARE
Copyright © 1994, Aspen Publishers, Inc.

Exhibit 4–10 Monthly Statistical Report

Referrals: Home Care _____ Month/year___________________

Hospice _____

Private Duty _____

Infusion _____

TOTAL _________

Discipline Breakdown:

SN_________

PT_________

OT_________

ST_________

MSS_________

AIDE_________

Homemaker_________

Companion _________

Psych Nursing ________________________

Case Management ____________________

Private Duty RN ______________________

Private Duty LPN _____________________

Private Duty NA ______________________

Pediatric _____________________________

Maternal _____________________________

Provider Breakdown:

Agency A _____ (Current_____ New referral_____)

Agency B _____ (Current_____ New referral_____)

Agency C _____ (Current_____ New referral_____)

Agency D _____ (Current_____ New referral_____)

Agency E _____ (Current_____ New referral_____)

Hospital Admissions:______________

Percentage referred to Home Care:______________

Submitted by:

____

Home Care Coordinator

Discharge Planning for Home Health Care
Copyright © 1994, Aspen Publishers, Inc.

◆ Appendix 4–A ◆

Criteria-Based Job Description and Evaluation: Home Care Coordinator

SYNOPSIS OF JOB FUNCTIONS

To develop timely, complete, appropriate, and individualized discharge plans for patients returning to the home setting based upon patient needs, psychosocial support systems, and financial support systems. To incorporate available community resources into the patient-centered home care referral.

Employee Name ______________________________ Date __________

Hire Date ______________________ Employee Number __________

Number of Years in This Position ______________________________

Evaluator's Name ______________________________

Evaluator's Title ______________________________

DISCHARGE PLANNING FOR HOME HEALTH CARE
Copyright © 1994, Aspen Publishers, Inc.

WORK ENVIRONMENT

Office and clinical work setting utilizes charts, files, and computers. Potential exposure to dust, fumes, smoke, gasses, talc, and other irritants.

WORK AIDS

Office supplies. Working knowledge of agency manuals. (HIM 11; Joint Commission standards; hospital administrative, human resource, infection control, Home Care Agency A departmental policy and procedures manuals). Working knowledge of American Nurses Association standards for nursing practice and acceptable standards of home care practice based upon available industry information.

EDUCATION AND EXPERIENCE

Licensed to practice professional nursing in the state of ________________________. B.S. in nursing or related field preferred. Minimum of 2 years of home care nursing and reimbursement knowledge required.

TRAITS

Ability to prioritize multiple demands. Organizational skills. Marketing skills. Motivated and a self-starter. Good interpersonal skills to communicate effectively with patients, families, hospital and departmental staff, and community agencies. Adheres to Joint Commission, Medicare, Medicaid, and other third party provider guidelines for planning posthospital care.

REQUIRED SAFETY NEEDS

Gloves, aprons, boots, masks, and gowns for appropriate clinical setting.

PHYSICAL DEMANDS

Lifting is not required beyond carrying of charts less than 10 pounds. Far vision correctable in one eye to 20/20 and 20/40 in the other eye. Specific vision needed: ability to read fine print. Specific hearing needed: ability to use a standard phone. Physical tasks include walking 2 hours, standing 2 hours, and sitting 4 hours. Hand dexterity needed for filing and documentation of work.

Discharge Planning for Home Health Care
Copyright © 1994, Aspen Publishers, Inc.

JOB RELATIONSHIPS

Reports directly to ____.

RATING SCALE TERMINOLOGY

1. *Excellent:* Often goes well beyond expectations of the job and has developed a cost-effective, efficient method that is incorporated into daily practice
2. *Commendable:* As a self-starter, puts forth a great deal of additional effort to consistently perform the functions of the job in an exemplary manner
3. *Good:* Meets all criteria of the job
4. *Improvement needed:* Inconsistent in job performance; does not meet all criteria of job
5. *Unsatisfactory:* Does not meet criteria of job; unable to perform job functions in an effective manner

JOB CRITERIA

Coordination of Home Care Referrals

1. Identifies potential home care needs of patients throughout the hospital.
   COMMENT: RATING:______________
2. Actively contributes in weekly departmental discharge planning meetings.
   COMMENT: RATING:______________
3. Thoroughly evaluates patient's medical, psychosocial, financial, and physical support systems to determine home care needs.
   COMMENT: RATING:______________
4. Collaborates with all members of the discharge planning team to promote an optimal plan for health care delivery in the home setting.
   COMMENT: RATING:______________
5. Communicates with the patient and family, if necessary, throughout the patient's hospitalization to elicit approval and support for the discharge plan.
   COMMENT: RATING:______________
6. Provides the patient with written information regarding patient rights and responsibilities and agency of patient's choice.
   COMMENT: RATING:______________

DISCHARGE PLANNING FOR HOME HEALTH CARE
Copyright © 1994, Aspen Publishers, Inc.

7. Negotiates with the physician in the development of the home care referral.
   COMMENT: RATING:______________
8. Provides a comprehensive home care referral at the time of hospital discharge to the agency of the patient's choice.
   COMMENT: RATING:______________
9. Follows the ______XYZ______ Hospital discharge plan and related intradepartmental policies and procedures.
   COMMENT: RATING:______________
10. Accurately verifies insurance coverage for home care and provides patient with a written evaluation of coverage after a complete explanation of benefits is given verbally.
    COMMENT: RATING:______________
11. Evaluates the cost effectiveness of alternative plans for the provision of health care.
    COMMENT: RATING:______________
12. Evaluates the records of all patients receiving Office of Aging custodial care before referral from the hospital in an attempt to identify unmet skilled needs.
    COMMENT: RATING:______________

Departmental/Professional Responsibilities

1. Participates in orientation of new personnel.
   COMMENT: RATING:______________
2. Participates in the development of new departmental goals and implementation of current goals.
   COMMENT: RATING:______________
3. Collaborates with other departmental personnel in the formation and revision of discharge planning process policies and procedures.
   COMMENT: RATING:______________
4. Is a resource and positive role model for departmental and hospital personnel.
   COMMENT: RATING:______________
5. Identifies potential problems and takes a proactive approach to alleviate the problem.
   COMMENT: RATING:______________
6. Attempts to problem solve staff-related issues on a one-to-one basis.
   COMMENT: RATING:______________

Copyright © 1994, Aspen Publishers, Inc.

7. Makes sound decisions and knows rationale for decisions based on knowledge and experience.
COMMENT: RATING:____________

8. Completes daily quality improvement screening information and forwards to the director of the department in a timely manner.
COMMENT: RATING:____________

9. Participates on at least one departmental committee.
COMMENT: RATING:____________

10. Participates on the hospital utilization review committee.
COMMENT: RATING:____________

11. Consistently completes job assignments without supervision.
COMMENT: RATING:____________

12. Provides proper notification of absence and/or tardiness.
COMMENT: RATING:____________

13. Is dependable in attendance.
COMMENT: RATING:____________

14. Is responsible for personal development.
COMMENT: RATING:____________

15. Maintains current knowledge of Medicare and other third party reimbursement and regulations independently.
COMMENT: RATING:____________

Collaboration with Other Health Care Professionals

1. Promotes a positive image of the hospital through collaborative and communicative efforts with outside agency personnel.
COMMENT: RATING:____________

2. Communicates effectively with prompt follow-through.
COMMENT: RATING:____________

3. Maintains open lines of communication with all staff.
COMMENT: RATING:____________

4. Respects the patient's rights by offering a choice of providers and maintaining confidentiality and privacy.
COMMENT: RATING:____________

DISCHARGE PLANNING FOR HOME HEALTH CARE
Copyright © 1994, Aspen Publishers, Inc.

5. Participates in hospital staff orientation and provides inservices to staff throughout the hospital.
   COMMENT: RATING:______________

6. Communicates both verbally and in written form to all patient care areas with updates in criteria/regulations or to problem solve identified situations.
   COMMENT: RATING:______________

HOSPITAL CRITERIA

Provides a current copy of license to supervisor.	Yes_____	No_____
Current CPR card.	Yes_____	No_____
Annual fire and safety update.	Yes_____	No_____
Annual Right To Know update.	Yes_____	No_____
Annual safety and body mechanics update.	Yes_____	No_____
Attends three job-related seminars/inservices.	Yes_____	No_____
Wears appropriate attire.	Yes_____	No_____
Wears hospital identification at all times.	Yes_____	No_____
Adheres to the philosophy and values of the hospital.	Yes_____	No_____

OVERALL RATING__________

EVALUATOR'S OVERALL COMMENTS:

EMPLOYEE'S COMMENTS:

____
Signature (optional)

DISCHARGE PLANNING FOR HOME HEALTH CARE
Copyright © 1994, Aspen Publishers, Inc.

◆ Chapter 5 ◆

The Social Work Perspective

ROLES AND RESPONSIBILITIES

The social worker focuses on the social framework and support systems available to the patient. These include the formal and informal systems: family and friends, as well as organized community resources. In today's world the social system includes both nuclear and augmented families, and the available community resources are often extensive.

The social worker is responsible for discussing with the patient, family, and support systems their unique social structure that provides the support needed for the patient at discharge. An analysis of the family's goals, power structure, values, culture, and expectations is necessary to determine the true posthospital patient/family picture.

Hospitalization is often unexpected, and the family and patient are in a crisis mode when the social worker first interacts with them. This initial interaction usually occurs within 24 hours of admission, at a time when posthospital care is often not a part of the patient's and family's thoughts. The social worker introduces this subject in a tactful, planned manner, and in fact the social worker's focus is the psychosocial and relationship factors, not the medical aspects of patient care.

Organizational placement of the social worker position is outlined in Chapter 4. The social worker within an institution can function as a consultant or in a direct service capacity. As a consultant, he or she serves as an educator to the health care team and as a communication link between the patient and physician. In the direct service capacity, he or she assesses the total situation and assists the patient and family to problem solve and communicate with each other. He or she becomes a patient advocate and is available to strengthen family support systems. The social worker offers alternatives of posthospital care to the patient.

The job description of the social worker position (Appendix 5–A) and Exhibits 5–1 through 5–5 are included to assist in the development or enhancement of the social worker role within your health care organization.

- *Social Work Referral Screen* (Exhibit 5–1): Used as a working tool; retained in the social work department files
- *Social Work Discharge Plan* (Exhibit 5–2): Page 2 of the referral screen; the original is kept on the patient's chart, and the third copy is retained in the social work department files
- *Social Work Assessment* (Exhibit 5–3): A screening tool utilized by the social worker when evaluating the patient; the original is retained in the social work department files, one copy is kept in the inpatient record, and one copy goes to the physician
- *Home Medical Equipment Work Sheet* (Exhibit 5–4): Physician orders for equipment; the original is sent to the equipment company, copy 1 is kept in the inpatient record, and copy 2 is kept in the social work department files (for current home medical equipment reimbursement criteria, see Appendix E)
- Monthly Statistical Report (Exhibit 5–5): Used to report statistical information to the department head and administration; retained on file in the social work department office

CANDIDATE SELECTION PROCESS

In your candidate search, an individual with qualifications similar to those of the home care coordinator should be sought. Exhibit 5–6 is a checklist to review the qualifications of social work applicants. Exhibit 5–7 is a guide of suggested interview questions. Once the checklist and interview are completed for each applicant, a pro and con comparison of applicants should be undertaken with prioritization of the attributes of each candidate.

A thorough knowledge of their peers and the group process in place within the organization assists the interviewer in the selection of a social worker who complements the discharge planning group.

Once candidates are prioritized, a reference check of the number 1 selection should be conducted and the hiring process completed.

Exhibit 5–1 Social Work Referral Screen

Date____________________

Patient Name ____________________

Address ____________________

Telephone ____________________

Birth date ____________________ Social Security number ____________________

Referral source ____________________ Referral date ____________________

Physician(s) ____________________ Diagnosis(es) ____________________

____________________ ____________________

____________________ ____________________

Surgery(ies) ____________________ Family contact(s) ____________________

____________________ ____________________

____________________ ____________________

Insurance information:

Medicare: ____________________

Medicaid: ____________________

Third party: ____________________

Other: ____________________

Income verification:

Income: ____________________ Source: ____________________

Other funds: ____________________ Source: ____________________

Social work service requested:

In hospital

_____Insurance verification

_____Medical assistance application

_____Counseling

_____Home visit/social work assessment (Exhibit 5–3)

_____Other: ____________________

____

____

Social service copy

DISCHARGE PLANNING FOR HOME HEALTH CARE
Copyright © 1994, Aspen Publishers, Inc.

Exhibit 5–2 Social Service Discharge Plan

Date_______________

Patient Name _______________

Address _______________

Telephone _______________

Birth date _______________ Social Security number _______________

Referral source _______________ Referral date _______________

Physician(s) _______________ Diagnosis(es) _______________

_______________ _______________

_______________ _______________

Surgery(ies) _______________ Family contact(s) _______________

_______________ _______________

_______________ _______________

Insurance information:

Medicare: _______________

Medicaid: _______________

Third Party: _______________

Other: _______________

Income verification:

Income: _______________ Source: _______________

Other funds: _______________ Source: _______________

Discharge plan/requested services

Home Care	*Extended Care*	*Discharge Summary*
Skilled nursing	Nursing home facility _______________	Transportation
Home health aide	Payment _______________	Yes_____ No_____
Therapy: _______________	Veterans hospital facility _______________	Arranged
Agency: _______________	Boarding home facility _______________	Source _______________
Equipment supplier (Exhibit 5–4)	Other _______________	Date _______________
Office of Aging	_______________	Other arrangements made:
Hospice		Transfer _______________
Meals on Wheels		Referral _______________
Other _______________		None needed _______________

Chart copy

DISCHARGE PLANNING FOR HOME HEALTH CARE
Copyright © 1994, Aspen Publishers, Inc.

Exhibit 5–3 Social Work Assessment

Patient Name: ____________________

Current address: ____________________

____________________ Phone: ____________________(H)

____________________ ____________________(W)

Birth date: ____________________

Date of admission: ____________________

Anticipated discharge date: ____________________

Admitting diagnosis(es): ____________________

____

Surgery(ies): ____________________

____

Insurance information: _____Medicare _____Medicaid

_____No known source _____Other ____________________

____

Verification: _____Yes _____No

____

Home environment: _____Home, alone _____Home, with spouse _____Home of relative

_____Other residents in home, specify

____

_____Facility name ____________________

_____No known place of residence

Resident assessment:

_____Family home _____# of floors

_____Apartment _____# of stairs

_____Mobile home

_____Multiple family home

Bathing facilities

Toilet _____Yes _____No _____Floor

Bath tub _____Yes _____No _____Floor

Shower _____Yes _____No _____Floor

Elevator _____Yes _____No

Other access _____Yes _____No Specify ____________________

____

Discharge Planning for Home Health Care
Copyright © 1994, Aspen Publishers, Inc.

Exhibit 5–3 continued

Transportation available: _____Car _____Taxi _____Bus

_____Other ______________________________

Activities of daily living: I = Independent D = Dependent

A = Assistance Needed

Bath_____ Dress_____ Stairs_____ Meal preparation_____

Toileting_____ Walking_____ Eating_____

Other ______________________________

Community resources utilized at time of admission:

_____Home health _____Veterans benefits _____Office of Aging

_____Nursing home _____Meals on Wheels _____Rehabilitative

_____HME ______Other, specify ______________________________

Patient/family identified/anticipated needs:

1. ______________________________
2. ______________________________
3. ______________________________

Potential to return home/or to prior situation:

Good_____ Fair_____ Poor_____

Anticipated health teaching needs: (per primary care nurse)

Diet_____	Patient_____	Family_____
Medications_____	Patient_____	Family_____
Procedures_____	Patient_____	Family_____
Treatments_____	Patient_____	Family_____
Other_____	Patient_____	Family_____

Equipment needs:

(per therapy/primary care nurse)

Walker_____ Cane_____ Wheelchair_____

Bed_____ O^2_____, specify ______________________________

Safety rails_____ Other_____

Patient needs care: Yes_____ No_____

Supervision: Yes_____ No_____

DISCHARGE PLANNING FOR HOME HEALTH CARE
Copyright © 1994, Aspen Publishers, Inc.

Exhibit 5–3 continued

Family/others available to provide support/care:

Yes_____ No_____

1. ____ Relationship ________________ Schedule _______

2. ____ Relationship ________________ Schedule _______

3. ____ Relationship ________________ Schedule _______

Alternate plan of care: ____

____

____

Social worker signature: ____

Date:______________________________

Copy: Yellow—Chart
White—Social work office files
Pink—Physician

Discharge Planning for Home Health Care
Copyright © 1994, Aspen Publishers, Inc.

Exhibit 5–4 Home Medical Equipment Work Sheet

Date:________________

Please note the identified needs for your patient. If you are in agreement, please sign as noted.

Physician signature: ________________

Date: ________________

Name: ________________

Room number: ________________

Home medical equipment needs:	Yes	No
Orthopedic needs:		
Walker		
Bedside commode		
Transfer board		
Cane, type		
Other, specify		
Other, specify		
Respiratory needs:		
Concentrator		
Liquid oxygen		
Monitor		
Ventilator		
Other, specify		
Comfort/personal needs:		
Bed		
Rails		
Trapeze		
Wheelchair		
Disposables, specify		
Other, specify		
Other, specify		

Original—Equipment company
Yellow copy—Record
Pink copy—Department

DISCHARGE PLANNING FOR HOME HEALTH CARE
Copyright © 1994, Aspen Publishers, Inc.

Exhibit 5–5 Monthly Statistical Report

	JAN	FEB	MARCH	APRIL	MAY	JUNE	JULY	AUG	SEPT	OCT	NOV	DEC	TOTAL YTD
Total inpatient admissions:													
• Adult M/S													
• OB/NBN													
• Pediatrics													
• Mental health													
• Rehab													
• Other													
Financial class breakdown:													
• Medicare													
• Medicaid													
• Self-pay													
• Other ________ ________ ________													
Total outpatient surgeries:													
• Adult M/S													
• Pediatrics													
Referral source screening criteria:													
• Physician													
• Nurse													
• Rehab therapist													

DISCHARGE PLANNING FOR HOME HEALTH CARE
Copyright © 1994, Aspen Publishers, Inc.

Exhibit 5–5 continued

	JAN	FEB	MARCH	APRIL	MAY	JUNE	JULY	AUG	SEPT	OCT	NOV	DEC	TOTAL YTD
• Utilization review													
• Emergency department													
• Outpatient surgery													
• Discharge conferences													
• PAT													
Actual patients screened:													
• No need													
• Need													
Posthospital care provided													
• HME													
1. Respiratory													
2. Orthopedic													
3. Other													
• Home health													
1. Medicare													
2. Third party													
3. Medicaid													
4. Self													
5. Other													
• ECF													
• SNF													
• Rehab center													
• Veterans facility													
ALOS													

DISCHARGE PLANNING FOR HOME HEALTH CARE
Copyright © 1994, Aspen Publishers, Inc.

Exhibit 5–6 Social Work Qualification Checklist

Is the candidate:	*Yes*	*No*	*Potential*
1. Master's prepared?			
2. Experienced?			Length of time:______
Acute care			
Long-term care			
Specialty			
Community			
Other, specify:			
3. Professional?			
Attire			
Verbal			
Nonverbal			
4. Equipped with strong communication skills?			
Verbal			
Written			
5. Knowledgeable of standards?			
Medicare			
Medicaid			
Joint Commission			
PRO			
Other, specify			
6. Knowledgeable of role of multidisciplinary team members?			
PT			
OT			
ST			
Dietitian			
Physician			
Nurse			
Pastoral care			
Administration			
Other, specify			
Availability date:			

DISCHARGE PLANNING FOR HOME HEALTH CARE
Copyright © 1994, Aspen Publishers, Inc.

Exhibit 5–7 Social Work Interview Questions

1. Describe your background as you believe it relates to this position. Describe how your usual day at work is spent.
2. Why are you seeking to change positions at this time? Is your boss aware that you are interviewing for this position? How will your resignation be received?
3. What are your 5-year, 10-year career goals? How do you expect to accomplish these goals?
4. What are your strengths as related to this position?
5. What are your weaknesses, in your perception, as they relate to this position?
6. Describe yourself using five adjectives your friends might use.
7. What activities do you participate in besides your work?
8. Describe your best prior work experience. What achievement are you most proud of in this position? What were your two most important responsibilities?
9. Describe your least liked prior work experience. What were you able to achieve in this position?
10. What knowledge and ability do you see that you need for this position? How would you obtain these?
11. Give two examples of the most difficult decisions you have made.
12. Is written or verbal communication most important in this type of position? Give two examples that demonstrate your ability with this type of communication.
13. Have you ever had to discipline an employee? How did you handle this situation? If you could redo this, would you handle it any differently? If so, what would you do?
14. Describe whom you currently report to in your present position. How does this boss interact with you? Is this one of your favorite bosses? If not, describe how you like a boss to interact with you.
15. Are you a success? Why do you believe this?
16. Describe how you would present a new idea to your boss. If this was approved, how would you implement it? If it was not approved, what would your next step be?
17. Individualize the situation.
18. Individualize the situation.
19. Individualize the situation.
20. Individualize the situation.

DISCHARGE PLANNING FOR HOME HEALTH CARE
Copyright © 1994, Aspen Publishers, Inc.

◆ Appendix 5–A ◆

Criteria-Based Job Description and Evaluation, Medical Social Worker

Position: Medical Social Worker

Employee Name:____

Employment date: ______________________________________

Last evaluation date: ___________________________________

Current evaluation date: ________________________________

Appraiser:______________________Signature: ____________________

Title: ________________________Date: _______________________

SYNOPSIS OF JOB FUNCTIONS

The medical social worker's primary function is to ensure continuity of care from the hospital into the posthospital care period. The social worker addresses the psychosocial and support system needs of the patient by providing ongoing one-on-one interactions throughout the hospitalization. Facilitation of the posthospital plan of care is accomplished via the merger of the social worker's knowledge of human behavior, values, culture, and social systems with his or her knowledge of the available community resources.

Discharge Planning for Home Health Care
Copyright © 1994, Aspen Publishers, Inc.

PERFORMANCE EXPECTATIONS

Direct Care Responsibilities

Assessment

1. Conducts chart review of 100 percent of identified high-risk patients within two (2) working days of admission. Rating_____
2. Meets with all appropriate high-risk patients within three (3) working days of admission. Rating_____
3. Conducts face-to-face assessments of all patients referred to the social services department within two (2) working days of referral. Rating_____
4. Completes a social work intake referral work sheet, which includes the following (see Exhibit 5–3):
   - history
   - personality style
   - family structure
   - ethnic/cultural background
   - basic coping mechanisms
   - interests
   - psychosocial factors
   - economic status
   - unique rehabilitation factors
   - special problems Rating_____
5. Identifies appropriate community resources currently being utilized by family/patient. Rating_____
6. Lists potential community resources available for specific patient needs. Rating_____
7. Actively participates in discharge planning meetings to identify potential patients with posthospital care problems. Rating_____

Planning/Implementation

1. Identifies the individual's potential posthospital care problems. Rating_____
2. Documents social work involvement on a regular basis. Rating_____
3. Identifies alternative solutions to posthospital care. Rating_____
4. Prepares forms and obtains necessary signatures for appropriate placements, such as (see Exhibit 5–2):

DISCHARGE PLANNING FOR HOME HEALTH CARE
Copyright © 1994, Aspen Publishers, Inc.

- skilled nursing homes
- veterans hospitals
- rehabilitation facilities
- extended care setting
- personal care setting
- group home setting Rating_____

5. Makes community referrals in a timely and comprehensive fashion. Rating_____
6. Assists families and patients with transfer and placement. Rating_____
7. Carries out discharge plan with attention to details. Rating_____
8. Records statistical data on a monthly basis (see Exhibit 5–5). Rating_____

Evaluation

1. Follows up posthospitalization via:
   - on-site visit
   - telephone call
   - patient/family survey Rating_____
2. Summarizes results of evaluations quarterly. Rating_____
3. Reviews quarterly results annually and uses results in annual report and revision of discharge plan. Rating_____
4. Annually reviews and makes appropriate revision of social work forms. Rating_____

Multidisciplinary Team Responsibilities

1. Maintains ongoing communication channels with appropriate health team members, such as:
   - physician
   - home care coordinator
   - physical therapist
   - occupational therapist
   - speech pathologist
   - utilization management
   - quality assurance/quality improvement
   - dietitian
   - pastoral care
   - administration
   - finance department

Rating_____

DISCHARGE PLANNING FOR HOME HEALTH CARE
Copyright © 1994, Aspen Publishers, Inc.

2. Communicates to appropriate health care team members final posthospital care plan. Rating_____

3. Responds in a timely fashion to social work consultant areas of the facility, such as:
    - outpatient surgery
    - primary care
    - ambulatory care
    - emergency care Rating_____

4. Demonstrates excellent verbal communication skills. Rating_____

Organizational Responsibilities

1. Participates actively on at least one (1) hospitalwide committee. Rating_____

2. Supervises social work student interns as assigned. Rating_____

3. Represents the health care organization within the community social work organization. Rating_____

4. Serves as a health care resource in areas such as:
    - community resources
    - psychosocial assessments
    - crisis intervention Rating_____

5. Demonstrates understanding and support of the health care organization's policies and procedures. Rating_____

6. Demonstrates knowledge and utilization of departmental policies and procedures. Rating_____

7. Applies social work principles and theories to the clinical setting. Rating_____

8. Serves as a patient advocate. Rating_____

9. Adheres to the principles of confidentiality in all aspects of his or her work. Rating_____

Evaluator's Comments: ____

____

____

____

____

DISCHARGE PLANNING FOR HOME HEALTH CARE
Copyright © 1994, Aspen Publishers, Inc.

Goals—Prior Year

1. ______________________________ Met____ Not Met____

2. ______________________________ Met____ Not Met____

3. ______________________________ Met____ Not Met____

4. ______________________________ Met____ Not Met____

5. ______________________________ Met____ Not Met____

Goals—Established for Current Year

____

____

____

____

____

Employee's Comments:

____

____

____

____

____

____

Employee Signature ______________________________

Date ______________________________

DISCHARGE PLANNING FOR HOME HEALTH CARE
Copyright © 1994, Aspen Publishers, Inc.

QUALIFICATIONS

1. Possess a Master's degree in social work from an accredited school of social work.
2. Demonstrates 1 year of recent social work experience, preferably in a similar health care setting.
3. Attends a minimum of two social work continuing education activities per year.
4. Maintains current health care standards of:

orientation	Yes_____	No_____
dress code	Yes_____	No_____
attendance	Yes_____	No_____
annual fire and safety update	Yes_____	No_____
annual infection control update	Yes_____	No_____
identification badge	Yes_____	No_____

5. Demonstrates excellent verbal and written communication skills.

WORKING ENVIRONMENT

Office and clinical work setting. Utilizes charts, files, and computers. Potential exposure to dust, fumes, smoke, or gas. Exposure to talc and other irritants.

WORKER TRAITS

Ability to organize work and to prioritize workload on an ongoing basis. Demonstrates initiative and creativity in meeting the posthospital care needs of patients and families. Adheres to Joint Commission, Medicare, Medicaid, and other third party provider guidelines for planning posthospital care.

PHYSICAL DEMANDS

Lifting is not required, carrying of charts less than 10 pounds. Far vision correctable in one eye to 20/20 and 20/40 in the other eye. Specific vision needed: ability to read fine print. Specific hearing needed: ability to use a standard telephone. Physical tasks include walking 4 hours, standing 2 hours, and sitting 2 hours. Hand dexterity needed for filing and documentation of work.

REQUIRED SAFETY NEEDS

Gloves, aprons, boots, masks, and gowns for appropriate clinical setting.

Reports directly to ____.

DISCHARGE PLANNING FOR HOME HEALTH CARE
Copyright © 1994, Aspen Publishers, Inc.

◆ Chapter 6 ◆

The Nursing Perspective

ROLES AND RESPONSIBILITIES

The hospital nurse plays an important role of patient advocate as he or she collaborates with other members of the discharge planning team. The nurse naturally spends the most time with patient and family interaction and therefore is the most logical person to assume the liaison role through the discharge planning process. Patient rapport begins to develop during the initial assessment and evaluation (Exhibit 3–2, Exhibit 6–1) leading to access of pertinent information about the patient. This information assists the team in developing the most realistic post discharge disposition. For example, the nurse not only communicates information about the patient's medical condition but also relays information about the authenticity of the support system and their ability to incorporate learning into practice. Much of what the nurse offers early in the discharge planning process becomes the framework for each individual plan.

Patients expect that they will either be taught to care for themselves or that the institution will arrange the necessary assistance to meet their needs beyond their in-patient stay. Responsibility for educating the patient and family falls predominantly on the nursing staff. Time expended in patient education is well worth the end results: enhanced customer satisfaction, minimized organizational liabilities and satisfied nursing staff as they meet their own needs to 'make a difference.' So often, health care workers forget that patients and families

Exhibit 6–1 Patient Initial Nursing Assessment

Patient Name: ______________________________

Chief Complaint: ______________________________

____

____

Physical (check if present)

EENT _____limited vision (_____L _____R)

_____glasses _____contacts

_____conjunctival discoloration

_____scleral discoloration _____pain

_____drainage _____PEARL

_____HOH (_____L _____R)

_____hearing aid (_____L _____R) _____drainage

_____pain

_____nasal passage blockage

_____deviant septum _____drainage

_____throat discoloration

_____swallowing difficulties

_____mouth ulcers _____mouth sores

_____gum edema _____edentulous

_____dentures (_____upper _____lower)

_____lymphadenopathy

Comments: ______________________________

____

____

____

Skin _____open areas _____scars _____dry _____oily

_____changes in pigmentation _____moles

Comments: ______________________________

____

____

____

DISCHARGE PLANNING FOR HOME HEALTH CARE
Copyright © 1994, Aspen Publishers, Inc.

Exhibit 6–1 continued

Neuromuscular ____alert ____oriented ____forgetful ____confused ____lethargic

____comatose ____tremors ____unsteady gait ____vertigo

____apprehensive ____hostile ____nonresponsive to pain

Comments: ____

____

____

____

Extremities

R arm ____normal ____weak ____flaccid ____contracture

L arm ____normal ____weak ____flaccid ____contracture

R leg ____normal ____weak ____flaccid ____contracture

L leg ____normal ____weak ____flaccid ____contracture

Comments: ____

____

____

____

Speech ____normal ____slurred ____aphasic

Language barrier ____Yes ____No

Comments: ____

____

____

____

Cardiac Pulse ____regular ____irregular ____apical rate ____radial rate

____extremity pulses + ____extremity pulses as normal

Blood pressure

	R	L
Lying		
Sitting		
Standing		

Discharge Planning for Home Health Care
Copyright © 1994, Aspen Publishers, Inc.

Exhibit 6–1 continued

Pain _____Yes _____No

Comments: ____

____

____

____

Pulmonary _____normal respirations

_____abnormal respirations

_____DOE _____Orthopnea _____CTA

_____abnormal aeration

_____respiratory rate

Comments: ____

____

____

____

Digestive _____active bowel sounds

_____abnormal bowel sounds

_____nausea _____vomiting _____diarrhea _____masses

_____constipation

_____special diet/fluid requirements

Comments: ____

____

____

____

Genitourinary _____frequency _____urgency _____dysuria

_____enuresis _____catheter _____pain

For men: _____date of last prostate exam

For women: _____date of last Pap smear

Comments: ____

____

____

____

Discharge Planning for Home Health Care
Copyright © 1994, Aspen Publishers, Inc.

Exhibit 6–1 continued

Musculoskeletal _____joint pain _____arthritis _____gout _____scoliosis _____lordosis
_____kyphosis _____back pain _____lymphadenopathy

Comments: ____

____

____

____

Current Medications

Name	*Dose*	*Frequency*	*Route*

Discussion occurred re: orientation to hospital room

_____patient rights/responsibilities

_____unit's daily routine _____primary nursing

_____patient's self-assessment

_____visiting hours/regulations _____identification band

Advance directives

_____patient provided verbal/written information

_____living will (patient _____has _____does not have)

_____do not resuscitate explanation

_____patient desires DNR

Discharge Planning for Home Health Care
Copyright © 1994, Aspen Publishers, Inc.

Exhibit 6–1 continued

____patient does not want DNR status

(____patient told to discuss with physician)

Name: ______________________________ Phone: ______________

Comments: ____

____

____

____

Valuables

Description	*Location*	
	Hospital Safe	*Patient Room*

RN Signature: ______________________________ Date: ______________

Retain as part of inpatient record

DISCHARGE PLANNING FOR HOME HEALTH CARE
Copyright © 1994, Aspen Publishers, Inc.

are lay people, without knowledge of the disease process, treatment procedure, and recovery time frames. What may be routine for the aide (giving a bath) may be overwhelming for the family. In these demanding times of efficiency, we must be careful not to forget effectiveness. Nurses are cautioned against assuming too much. The health care worker who states, "There is no need for home nursing because the wound only needs a wet to dry saline dressing" not only fails to meet the expectations of the patient and family but also the expectations of state and national regulatory bodies.

The third major role for the bedside nurse is to provide complete and accurate information to promote continuity of care. As the patient's condition changes from day to day, the observant nurse needs to communicate these changes to the rest of the team for the fine tuning of the discharge plan to occur. Time is of the essence; this information can be communicated by a written note in the patient record, informal verbal communication, or electronic mail. Regardless of the patient disposition, the health caregivers on the receiving end will require baseline data on referral forms. The organization that supplies accurate information develops a credible reputation. Failure to provide complete and accurate information when making a referral may result in discharge delays for your institution since outside providers more readily accept patients referred from a more reliable organization. For the patient returning home with home health care, comprehensive written discharge instructions (Exhibit 6–2) must be provided. It is imperative that the nurse be assertive in procurement of the needed information. Medication regimes frequently change during hospitalization; therefore, writing "Meds as before" is not sufficient. Knowing that faulty medication compliance is one of the major contributing factors of illness among our seniors, the nurse needs to intervene with the busy physician and get precise discharge medication orders. This also meets the needs of the agencies accepting patients referred from the organization. It is not possible to instruct a patient with a new medication regime without clear discharge orders.

Unfortunately, there are many adversities for the bedside nurse in fulfilling her discharge planning responsibilities. Rising patient acuity levels and dwindling staffing downgrades the importance of discharge planning activities. Discharge planning becomes low-man-on-the-totem pole. Tom Peters, a leading business consultant, emphasizes the need to listen to your customers. If we listen, patients and families are heard to complain of feeling isolated and having been discharged unprepared for self care. Nurses have voiced similar displeasure with lack of time to adequately provide their patient with advocacy and liaison activities. To rectify these system problems, the role of a Clinical Care Manager (CCM) is recommended.

The most effective Clinical Care Managers are senior nurses with a vast amount of clinical expertise and management experience. Organizations have the option of identifying the CCM's specialty area. Some have had success with assignment of CCMs to specific physicians while others assign their care managers to specific specialty areas such as neurology or oncology. Patient satisfaction inevitably rises as the Clinical Care Manager interacts with the patient from admission through discharge. The CCM serves as a positive role model and good resource for the unit staff nurses. Clinical and managerial experience of the CCM provides the ability to complete the role responsibilities including:

- *Liaison Activities*—Effective communication skills are essential for interaction with the various team members. The ability to negotiate win-win situations and advocate for patient needs is an essential function of this position.
- *Patient Education Activities*—This position has an opportunity to work closely with the patient and their significant others. Educating the patient about the disease process and post hospital care needs is a vital role and one that the CCM has time to complete.
- *Discharge Planning Activities*—Knowledge of community resources and a working knowledge of the various levels of care is an asset to the CCM as he or she evaluates the individual patient's status in relationship to the post discharge disposition. The CCM's input is immeasurable to the successful outcome for the patient.
- *Care Organization Activities*—The CCM follows the patient's progress with the clinical path and using excellent communication skills calls variations in the patient's progress to the attention of the appropriate team member. Informing and counseling the patient and significant others about their role in the patient's care contributes to the success of the path. (For sample diagnosis related discharge planning/instructional clinical care plans/clinical pathways, refer to Appendixes F, G, and H.)

A postdischarge follow-up phone call by the CCM provides the little extra that is necessary to exceed the patient's (customer) expectations. This also provides the organization with valuable input regarding the effectiveness of the posthospital plan. A sample phone interview questionnaire is provided in Exhibit 6–3.

The role of the nurse is pivotal in discharge planning. As a nursing administrator, regardless of whether your organization employs Clinical Care Managers or primary care nurses, you must advocate for nurse involvement with discharge planning. The valuable input the nurse receives during the course of his or her daily assignments helps to ensure that all patient needs will be met and that the most appropriate disposition will be planned.

Exhibit 6–2 Patient Discharge Instructions

Name: ______________________ Date: ______________

Address: ______________________________________

____

Accompanied by: ______________________ Relationship: ______________

____

Medications	*Dose*	*Times*	*Written Information Given* Yes	No

Diet: ______________________ Fluid requirements: ______________

Personalized instructions: ______________________________

____

____

Next physician visit:

Doctor______________ Appt.______________ Phone______________

Doctor______________ Appt.______________ Phone______________

Doctor______________ Appt.______________ Phone______________

Discharge Planning for Home Health Care
Copyright © 1994, Aspen Publishers, Inc.

Exhibit 6–2 continued

Referrals made to:

1) Agency ____ Phone ______________

Agency will contact patient by _____phone _____writing _____home visit

2) Agency ____ Phone ______________

Agency will contact patient by _____phone _____writing _____home visit

The following valuables were returned: ________________________________

____

____

____

I received a written copy of my discharge instructions after a verbal explanation. I understand these instructions.

________________________________ ________________________________

Patient/Designee Relationship

____

Date

Original—Patient
Copy—Patient record

DISCHARGE PLANNING FOR HOME HEALTH CARE
Copyright © 1994, Aspen Publishers, Inc.

Exhibit 6–3 Postdischarge Phone Interview

Patient name: ______________________________

Phone: ______________________ Diagnosis: ______________________

Discharge date: ______________________________

Today's date: ______________________________

1. *Current functional level*

Activity	*Independent*	*Requires Support*	*Identified Problem*
Ambulation			
Transfers			
Dressing/grooming			
Food preparation			
Eating			
Taking medication			

2. *Medications*

Did you get your prescriptions filled? Yes No

Do you have any questions about your:

medication schedule? Yes No

medication actions? Yes No

medication side effects? Yes No

Do you have any problems taking your medications? Yes No

Identified problems: ______________________________

____

____

____

3. *Sign and symptoms*

Do you have any symptoms? (relate to diagnosis) Yes No

If you are a surgical patient, is your incision dry without discoloration? Yes No

Discharge Planning for Home Health Care
Copyright © 1994, Aspen Publishers, Inc.

Exhibit 6–3 continued

Do you have any drainage? (specify)	Yes	No
Do you have a fever?	Yes	No

Identified problems: ____

____

____

____

4. *Follow-up*

Were you contacted by ____________________(agency)?	Yes	No
____________________(HME)?	Yes	No
Did you schedule a physician appointment?	Yes	No
Did you see the physician?	Yes	No
Are you getting the necessary help from:		
friends/family?	Yes	No
agencies?	Yes	No
other?	Yes	No

Instructions/referrals provided:

____

____

____

____

____

____

____

____

____

Discharge Planning for Home Health Care
Copyright © 1994, Aspen Publishers, Inc.

◆ Chapter 7 ◆

Professional Collaboration

OVERVIEW

To meet the total array of needs of the hospitalized patient and his or her family today, the interaction of health care providers from multiple disciplines is essential. These professionals should assess the patient thoroughly in their area of specialization and communicate unique and specific posthospital care needs to the patient's primary discharge planner.

Because patient needs frequently change, it is important to have a means for ongoing communication and updating of the patient's progress. A tool utilized for this purpose is the multidisciplinary discharge planning flow sheet (Exhibit 7–1).

Each of the treatment/health care modalities identified within the discharge planning process is an important contributor to the patient's posthospital care plan. The plan is only as strong and vital as each link in the process. Collaboration and communication among professionals serve as the fabric that holds together and gives texture to the discharge plan. Turf issues and professional competitiveness must take a back seat so that true collaborative discharge planning can be accomplished. In today's world, where the time factor figures prominently in the patient's posthospital care plan, positive efforts by all professionals to contribute to the total discharge plan of the patient are vital. This chapter elaborates on the individual role of each professional in the discharge planning process.

THE PHYSICIAN

The role of the physician in discharge planning is pivotal to the success of the plan. The physician alone possesses the knowledge of the complexities of the patient's condition and needs to communicate these complexities and any unique medical care-related needs to the discharge planning team. When a home health follow-up is indicated, there needs to be significant dialogue between the hospital home care coordinator and the patient's physician. All physicians and surgeons involved in patient care should contribute to the patient's discharge plan. The primary physician for follow-up care, however, should be the physician or surgeon who oversees the primary posthospitalization plan of care.

The physician is the health care professional who admits and discharges the patient. It is he or she who prescribes the posthospital treatment plan and facilitates communication among the family, patient, multidisciplinary team, and support systems.

It is vital that the physician document the inpatient treatment plan and anticipated discharge date early in the patient's hospital course so that all the links in the discharge planning chain can be consulted for input.

The physician needs to focus beyond the acute medical / surgical condition to the socioeconomic setting of the patient and must determine, initially, whether a return to the previous living condition is possible for the patient. The family physician who has been providing ongoing care to the family is best equipped to assist in this determination.

As the patient or family / support system conditions change, it is important that the family, patient, and physician communicate these changes. Conversely, other team members must apprise the physician of changing conditions; a well-informed multidisciplinary team is able to keep up to date on the patient's needs. The multidisciplinary team is available to assist the physician in the assessment areas needed for comprehensively planning posthospital care.

THE UTILIZATION MANAGEMENT SPECIALIST

The utilization management specialist reviews and monitors hospital length of stay and correlates these statistics with Medicare, Medicaid, and peer review organization denials and reconsiderations (Exhibit 7–2). These statistics are shared in hospitalwide utilization management meetings, where denial trends (Exhibit 7–3) are identified for support of prompt discharge planning.

These individuals develop criteria and perform concurrent screening and monitoring of charts to determine compliance with regulations and assurance of reimbursement by third party payors. Documentation is reviewed for appropriateness and reimbursement ability.

When indicated, precertification reviews are conducted, and length of stay is preapproved for reimbursement. Ongoing prior approval is obtained for cases that extend beyond accepted lengths of stay.

Specifically identified placement problems are evaluated for appropriateness and level of care needs and are summarized in a utilization management work sheet (Exhibit 7–4).

Exhibit 7–1 Multidisciplinary Discharge Planning Flow Sheet

Name: ____________________

Room: ____________________

Name/discipline	Date/time	Need identified	Follow-up	Completed

Abbreviation legend:

- DDS—dentist
- DO, MD—physician
- HHCC—hospital home care coordinator
- LPN,RN—nursing
- OT—occupational therapy
- PA—physician's assistant
- PC—pastoral care
- PT—physical therapy
- QA—quality assurance specialist
- RD—registered dietitian
- RT—respiratory therapy
- ST—speech therapy
- SW—social work
- UR—utilization review specialist

DISCHARGE PLANNING FOR HOME HEALTH CARE
Copyright © 1994, Aspen Publishers, Inc.

Exhibit 7–2 Utilization Management Monthly/Year-to-Date Summary

DATA	JAN	FEB	MAR	APR	MAY	JUNE	JULY	AUG	SEP	OCT	NOV	DEC	YTD	COMMENTS
Total admissions														
Total ALOS														
• M/S														
• OB/NBN														
• Rehab														
• MH														
Reviews completed														
• Concurrent														
• Admission														
• Retrospective														
Inquires completed														
Total inpatient stays (14 days or over)														
• M/S														
• Rehab														
• MH														
Admission financial class data total														
• Medicare														
• Medicaid														
• Self-pay														
• Blue Cross														
• CHAMPUS														
• Other third party														

Retain in department files

DISCHARGE PLANNING FOR HOME HEALTH CARE
Copyright © 1994, Aspen Publishers, Inc.

Exhibit 7–3 Utilization Management Denial Trends

					JAN	FEB	MAR	APR	MAY	JUNE	JULY	AUG	SEP	OCT	NOV	DEC	YTD	COMMENTS
Denials		TOTAL:																
Type	DRG	Charges	LOS															
Denials pending		TOTAL:																
Type	DRG	Charges	LOS															
Denials reversed		TOTAL:																
Type	DRG	Charges	LOS															

Retain in department files

Copyright © 1994, Aspen Publishers, Inc.

Exhibit 7–4 Utilization Management Work Sheet

Patient Name ______________________________ DRG ______________

Room number ______________________________ LOS ______________

Outlier days ______________

Complications ______________

Level of care

_____Acute—new illness, critical stages

_____Skilled—ongoing skilled care needed

_____Intermediate— restorative care needs
patient semi–self-sufficient
probable home placement _____Yes _____No

_____Custodial— needs ADL assistance
probable long-term duration
plateaued

Facility needed

_____Skilled nursing facility—AVAILABILITY ______________________________

_____Extended care facility—AVAILABILITY ______________________________

_____Group homes

_____Personal care homes

_____Veterans hospital

_____Rehabilitation center

_____Mental health

_____Retirement home

_____Other, specify ______________________________

Action Plan for Expedited Discharge

What	*Who*	*Where*	*Follow-up*

Retain in department files

DISCHARGE PLANNING FOR HOME HEALTH CARE
Copyright © 1994, Aspen Publishers, Inc.

Exhibit 7–5 Utilization Management Average Length of Stay Summary

Fiscal year______________

JAN	FEB	MAR	APR	MAY	JUN	JUL	AUG	SEP	OCT	NOV	DEC	
												14.00
												13.75
												13.50
												13.25
												13.00
												12.75
												12.50
												12.25
												12.00
												11.75
												11.50
												11.25
												11.00
												10.75
												10.50
												10.25
												10.00
												9.75
												9.50
												9.25
												9.00
												8.75
												8.50
												8.25
												8.00
												7.75
												7.50
												7.25
												7.00
												6.75
												6.50
												6.25
												6.00
												5.75
												5.50
												5.25
												5.00
												4.75
												4.50
												4.25
												4.00
												3.75
												3.50
												3.25
												3.00
												2.75
												2.50
												2.25
												2.00

Retain in department files

Discharge Planning for Home Health Care
Copyright © 1994, Aspen Publishers, Inc.

These specialists historically have focused predominantly on Medicare and Medicaid patients, but their role is expanding in the tightly controlled health care reform of today. The utilization management specialist determines the number of expected days of hospitalization for the patient in light of the patient's diagnosis, hospital treatment course, and any complicating factors. The specialist notifies the physician and patient when the course of stay will no longer be financed by third party payors.

The overall average length of stay has become a key index of the hospital's fiscal viability. It has become the responsibility of the Utilization Management department to maintain a current hospitalwide graph of the hospital's total average length of stay on a monthly basis (Exhibit 7–5).

Utilization management specialists must use foresight in the anticipation of barriers to patients' discharges to maintain these length of stays at an acceptable level. Their contribution to the patient's discharge planning meeting often provides time frame guidelines that help organize the planning process.

QUALITY ASSURANCE/QUALITY IMPROVEMENT

The role of this specialist is to identify quality issues within the discharge planning process and to monitor this process for compliance with established thresholds. Indicators are developed that are measurable on both concurrent and retrospective modes. One example of a discharge planning quality improvement indicator that can be reviewed concurrently is the readmission rate; Exhibit 7–6 places this criterion in an acceptable format for the Joint Commission on Accreditation of Healthcare Organizations. Other examples of discharge planning quality improvement indicators are listed on the discharge planning daily screening checklist (Exhibit 7–7). These can be developed in a format similar to that for the readmission rate criteria.

In addition to ongoing daily monitoring, this specialist should conduct follow-up patient satisfaction surveys at least quarterly to determine the patients' and families' general level of satisfaction with the discharge planning process. Additionally, retrospective reviews of actual discharge records should be conducted to determine the level of compliance with discharge planning teaching within the institution.

There are multitudinous examples of criteria to establish and review in the area of discharge planning; several are as follows:

- *Discharge planning documentation*
  1. initiated upon admission
  2. high-risk cases reviewed within 24 hours of discharge
  3. multidisciplinary involvement appropriate and documented
  4. ongoing efforts documented at least weekly
- *Overstays reviewed at least every 48 hours*

Exhibit 7–6 Quality Assurance/Quality Improvement Indicator

Scope of care: Discharge planning

Aspect of care monitored: Readmission

Indicator: Inappropriate admissions/readmissions can be prevented by comprehensive discharge planning

Threshold for evaluation: 90 percent

Sample: 100 percent of all readmissions within 7, 14, and 30 days are evaluated

Methodology: The admission registrar reviews all admission/readmission statistics on a daily basis, and data collected are forwarded on a daily screening sheet (Exhibit 7–7) to the quality assurance specialist for analysis

Data source: Admission registration list, discharge list

Data collectors: Quality assurance/quality improvement specialist
Medical record clerk
Admissions registrar

Original—QA/QI manual

Copyright © 1994, Aspen Publishers, Inc.

Exhibit 7–7 Discharge Planning Daily Screening Checklist

Date: ____________________

Involved Employee Number: ____________________

Patient Number: ____________________

Indicator Reason

1. Readmits within 30 days
   _____Hospital
   _____LTC
   _____Emergency department
2. Incidents
   _____Patient
   _____Staff
3. Patient/family perception of discharge planning services
   _____Dissatisfaction expressed
      _____Verbal
      _____Written
      _____Questionnaire feedback
4. Preadmission planning
   _____Discharge not completed
   _____Misinformation
   _____Forgotten/late referral
5. Facility complaints
   Facility ____________________
6. Unexpected death

Explanation/Action: ____________________

____

____

____

REPORTED BY: ____________________ DATE: ____________________

Retain in department files

DISCHARGE PLANNING FOR HOME HEALTH CARE
Copyright © 1994, Aspen Publishers, Inc.

- *Discharge teaching is:*
  1. initiated a minimum of 24 hours before discharge
  2. accurate
- *Comprehensive discharge teaching implemented, to include as appropriate:*
  1. medications
  2. treatments
  3. community resources
  4. diet instruction
  5. follow-up care provider information
  6. other (specify)

All criteria screened and evaluated should then be summarized in a monthly report (Exhibit 7–8) with a monitoring log (Exhibit 7–9) for those criteria that fall below the established thresholds.

THE RESPIRATORY THERAPIST

One role that is often overlooked for participation on the discharge planning team is the respiratory therapist. This person has developed a rapport with the patient while spending hours at the bedside providing breathing treatments and instructions to promote the exchange of gases. Ease of breathing is a vital need, and the help given by the respiratory therapist often enhances patient/family rapport.

For the patient returning to the home setting, the respiratory therapist evaluates the layout of the patient's home and recommends specific types of oxygen equipment based upon the patient's usage. His or her knowledge of equipment and oxygen costs as well as reimbursement criteria of third party payors must be current. For example, Medicare currently requires an oxygen saturation level below 89 percent for oxygen to be a covered expense for a patient with chronic obstructive pulmonary disease. Medicare also will not reimburse for oxygen as needed but will cover oxygen if ordered up to 24 hours per day. It is helpful for the respiratory therapist to alert the home care coordinator of the specific respiratory-related equipment being ordered and then to make the referral directly to the respiratory therapist at the home medical equipment company.

In some instances patients require specific, detailed respiratory-related instructions. These are best provided by the respiratory therapist. This person is responsible for initiating the instructions and documenting the patient's learning response and status at the time of discharge. Specifics can be relayed via communication forms such as the interdepartmental communication sheet (see Exhibit 4–7) or by informal verbal communication.

Exhibit 7–10 is a sample instructional care plan that could be put onto carbonless copy paper so that a copy could be sent with the home care referral. The respiratory therapist should also attend family conferences and patient discharge planning meetings when the complicated patient situation necessitates continued respiratory care after hospitalization.

Exhibit 7–8 Discharge Planning Quality Assurance/Quality Improvement Monthly Summary

MONTH/YEAR ____________

Indicator	*Findings*	*Action*
INDICATOR: Threshold ____________		
Compliance ____________		
INDICATOR: Threshold ____________		
Compliance ____________		
INDICATOR: Threshold ____________		
Compliance ____________		

File in department's QA/QI manual

Copyright © 1994, Aspen Publishers, Inc.

Exhibit 7–9 Discharge Planning Quality Assurance/Quality Improvement Indicator Summary Log

Date:____________________

Initial Reporting Date	*Indicator Evaluated*	*Reevaluation Date*	*Results*	*Current Action*	*Proposed Action*	*Additional Follow-up*	*Date*

File in department's QA/QI manual

Discharge Planning for Home Health Care
Copyright © 1994, Aspen Publishers, Inc.

THE PHYSICAL THERAPIST

The physical therapist also interacts closely with the patient, which allows him or her to offer specific recommendations based upon his or her expertise. Physical therapists are responsible for evaluating the patient's physical capabilities in conjunction with the disease process, for developing a plan of care directed toward achievement of individualized goals, and for recommending specific follow-up care for the physician's approval. Frequently, it is the physical therapist who discusses the patient's unrealistic expectations and assists the patient to identify the adaptation methods that meet the reality of his or her physical condition. The astute physical therapist talks with family members and discovers what home modifications are required before discharge. Working closely with the family provides the therapist an opportunity to educate the patient's support system about the specific needs after discharge that will ensure a viable plan.

The physical therapist must also communicate needs to the home care coordinator if the patient is returning home or to the social worker if the patient is going to a skilled nursing facility or rehabilitation facility. The information the physical therapist provides should become a part of the referral work sheet for transmission to the receiving physical therapist. Although there is value in different professionals evaluating the same patient, the information provided by the hospital therapist offers a baseline and promotes continuity of care.

Exhibit 7–11 is one example of a physical therapy status and evaluation form. A copy of this form would be helpful to the receiving therapist. Physical therapists often provide a wealth of information in discharge planning unit meetings and family conferences, especially during the provision of acute rehabilitation, and they should make every effort to attend these meetings.

THE OCCUPATIONAL THERAPIST

The occupational therapist is the discharge planning team member who, being cognizant of the patient's altered self-concept in relationship to activities of daily living and the patient's dependency upon others, evaluates the effects of disease on the patient's ability to bathe, groom, prepare nourishment, clean, return to the workforce, and complete other aspects of daily care. In helping the patient adapt, the occupational therapist provides the patient with an outlet to verbalize apprehensions and disappointments. As the occupational therapist educates the patient and family, he or she helps the patient reach maximum potential toward highly individualized goals. Often, the patient's motivational force lies within the patient's desire to resume activities of daily living.

Family conferences and patient discharge planning meetings benefit by the presence of the occupational therapist. Realistic goals and time frames help the team reach difficult decisions, such as where to go after the hospital, what to expect, and when it will happen. Exhibit 7–12 is an occupational therapy status and evaluation form that, when forwarded to the receiving occupational therapist, provides necessary communication to aid in continuity of

Exhibit 7–10 Respiratory Therapy Infant CPR Instruction Sheet

Patient Name ______________________ Parent Name 1 ______________________

Room # ______________________ Parent/Designee Name 2 ______________________

	Initial		*Follow-up*		
Instructional Step	*Provided by*	*Provided on (Date)*	*Recall Obtained on*	*Reinstruction Provided on*	*By Independent Demonstration*
1. Disease process					
2. Signs/symptoms (when to begin CPR)					
3. Locating brachial pulse					
4. Continuing brachial pulse					
5. Assessing respiratory rate					
6. Assessing airway patency					
7. Positioning infant for CPR					
8. Cardiac compressions					
• positioning of fingers					
• depth					
• frequency					
9. Respirations					
• positioning of mouth					
• amount of air					
• frequency					
10. Reassessing status					
• frequency					
• when to stop					
11. Need for certified course					
Date					
Place					

Retain in patient record

Discharge Planning for Home Health Care
Copyright © 1994, Aspen Publishers, Inc.

Exhibit 7–11 Physical Therapy Status and Evaluation Form

Patient Name: ______________________________

Room #: ______________________ Date: ______________

Diagnosis: ______________________ Date of onset: ______________

Current status:

Behavioral: ______________________ Mental: ______________

Strength: RUE: ______________________ LUE: ______________

RLE: ______________________ LLE: ______________

Range of motion/reflexes: RUE: ______________________

LUE: ______________________

RLE: ______________________

LLE: ______________________

Transferability: Bed mobility: ______________________

Supine to sit: ______________________

Sit to stand: ______________________

Wheelchair: ______________________

Gait: Steady ______________ Ataxic ______________ Stairs ______________

Other (explain) ______________________

Assistive device ______________________

Balance: Sitting ______________________

Standing ______________________

Plan of Care	*Goals*	*Status*

Disposition: Rehab facility_____ SNF_____ ICF_____ Personal care_____ Home_____

If home, describe setting: ______________________________

____

____

Patient signature: ______________________

Original—patient record
Copy 1—department record
Copy 2—receiving PT

DISCHARGE PLANNING FOR HOME HEALTH CARE
Copyright © 1994, Aspen Publishers, Inc.

patient care. Exhibit 7–13 can be utilized by either the physical therapist or the occupational therapist in evaluation of the home to assist with developing the plan of care and the discharge plan.

Like members of other disciplines, the occupational therapist must communicate his or her actions and recommendations for the patient's discharge either via the interdepartmental communication sheet (see Exhibit 4–7) or through verbal methods. Information must be written into the patient's record for dissemination and legal purposes.

THE SPEECH THERAPIST

The speech therapist evaluates the patient's ability to communicate and implements an individualized plan of care designed to meet realistic patient goals. As a part of the discharge planning team, the speech therapist should communicate his or her recommendation via the interdepartmental communication form (see Exhibit 4–7). His or her expertise is essential in family conferences and patient discharge planning meetings because communication skills are an essential component of patient safety. Exhibit 7–14 is an example of a speech therapy assessment form that will help ensure continuity of care.

THE DIETITIAN

Poor nutrition is a major social and health issue in the United States, contributing to disease onset and progression. The dietitian is the professional who provides patient education regarding specialized diets. This important role should not be overlooked. Intervention should occur early in the patient's hospitalization and should utilize the learning process steps outlined in Chapter 3. The patient must be given:

- time to absorb new information
- time to review written instructions
- time to ask questions
- information to incorporate cultural foods into his or her special diet

The dietitian is of the most appropriate discipline to evaluate the patient's financial, cultural, and eating patterns that affect his or her special diet. When the cook is someone other than the patient, he or she should have the opportunity to obtain complete instructions about the meal plan. All educational and evaluative actions must be documented in the patient record and verbalized to the Home Care Coordinator before the hospital discharge. Exhibit 7–15 may be used by the dietitian as a work sheet during the patient's hospitalization.

Exhibit 7–12 Occupational Therapy Status and Evaluation Form

Name: ______________________ Date: ______________

Room #: ______________________

Diagnosis: ______________________ Date of onset: ______________

Current status:

Behavioral ______________ Motivation ______________

Stress level ______________ Marital ______________

Cognition ______________ Memory ______________

Strength: RUE ______________ LUE ______________

ROM: RUE ______________ LUE ______________

HDL ability:

Bathing ______________________

Grooming ______________________

Dressing ______________________

Meal prep ______________________

Use of phone ______________________

Use of money ______________________

Use of appliances ______________________

Work hardening:

Position immediately preceding ______________________

Required tasks to return ______________________

____

____

Expectation for return ______________________

Plan of Care	*Goals*

Disposition: Rehab facility____ SNF____ ICF____ Personal care____ Home____

OT Signature ______________________

Date ______________________

Original—inpatient record
Copy 1—department files
Copy 2—receiving therapist

DISCHARGE PLANNING FOR HOME HEALTH CARE
Copyright © 1994, Aspen Publishers, Inc.

Exhibit 7–13 Home Assessment Form

Patient Name: ______________________________

Address: ______________________________

Date of Assessment: ______________________________

By: ____________________ Title: ____________________

External Conditions

Type of dwelling: apartment_____ 1-floor single_____ 2-floor single_____
2-floor duplex_____ elevator_____

Entrance: # of steps_____ width of steps_____ railing_____ (1-side L/R) (both sides)
Door: Width _____inches, opens to L/R

Fire escape: Yes No Location ______________________________

Utilities

Type of heat: ______________________________

Phone: Type ______________________________
Number ______________________________
Location ______________________________

Type of appliances: stove/oven ______________________________

Electricity: Yes No Running water: Yes No Hot Cold

Rooms

Kitchen

Door width _____inches

Floor material ______________________________

Diagram of room: 1 square = 1 foot

Discharge Planning for Home Health Care
Copyright © 1994, Aspen Publishers, Inc.

Exhibit 7–13 continued

Cabinets: Height from floor _____inches

Counter tops: Height from floor _____inches

Bathroom

Door width _____inches

Toilet height _____inches

Bath tub height _____inches

Shower: Yes No Handheld: Yes No

Wall material ______________________ Can grab bars be added? Yes No

Floor material ______________________

Diagram of room: 1 square = 1 foot

Living Room

Door width _____inches

Type of furniture ______________________

Height of furniture: Sofa_____ Chair 1_____ Chair 2_____ Chair 3_____

Floor material ______________________

Bedrooms	#1	#2	#3
Door width			
Size of room			
Type of bed			
Height of bed			
Type of closet			

DISCHARGE PLANNING FOR HOME HEALTH CARE
Copyright © 1994, Aspen Publishers, Inc.

Exhibit 7–13 continued

Hallway width ______inches (1st floor)

______inches (2nd floor)

Transportation available: Yes No

Type of vehicle ____

Driver name ______________________Relationship ______________________

Comments: Include information about patient's support system if available.

____

____

____

____

____

____

____

____

____

____

____

____

____

____

____

Signature ______________________________

Title ______________________________

Original—patient record
Copy 1—department files
Copy 2—receiving therapist

Discharge Planning for Home Health Care
Copyright © 1994, Aspen Publishers, Inc.

PASTORAL CARE

A member of the pastoral care team is available to all patients at any time. The on-call team member can be consulted when indicated to assist the patient and family in planning for posthospital care. The pastoral care team member enhances the multidisciplinary discharge team's understanding of the ethnic and emotional components of the family's dynamics that affect the discharge plan.

When the patient and family are faced with especially difficult decisions, the pastoral care team member is viewed as a neutral participant, able to lend support to the patient and family during these difficult times.

The individual's community pastor is welcome to participate in the discharge planning process when appropriate and can often offer additional insight into the patient and family dynamics being presented.

Independent of the consultant approach to pastoral care intervention, pastoral care screening criteria can be utilized upon admission to identify potential families and patients for whom pastoral care might prove to be an asset to the discharge planning process as well as to assist in meeting other posthospital care needs of the patient (Exhibit 7–16). The pastoral care team should be involved in all identified hospice referrals and should be consulted to meet with the patient and his or her family when they are facing referrals to the hospice program. Pastoral care is an excellent resource for church-related and other community assistance programs.

Exhibit 7–14 Speech Therapy Status and Evaluation Form

Patient Name: ______________________________ Date: ______________

Room #: ____

Diagnosis: ______________________________ Date of onset: __________

Patient lives: Alone____ With ____ others (specify)

____

____

____

Financial status: ______________________________________

Speech: Normal ______________________________________

Alaryngeal ______________________________________

Language barrier ________________________________

Deficit (specify) ________________________________

____

Swallowing: Normal ______________________________________

Dysphangia ____________ Diet ______________________

Home food preparation by ________________________

Blender available Yes____ No____

Reading: Normal ______________________________________

Deficit (specify) ________________________________

____

____

Comprehension ________________________________

Writing: Normal ______________________________________

Deficit (specify) ________________________________

____

Dominance L hand R hand

Discharge Planning for Home Health Care
Copyright © 1994, Aspen Publishers, Inc.

Exhibit 7–14 continued

Plan of Care	*Goals*	*Status*

Signature: ______________________________

Title ______________________________

Original—patient record
Copy 1—department files
Copy 2—receiving therapist

DISCHARGE PLANNING FOR HOME HEALTH CARE
Copyright © 1994, Aspen Publishers, Inc.

Exhibit 7–15 Dietitian Work Sheet

Patient Name: ______________________________ Room #: ______________

Diagnosis: ______________________________ Date of onset: ______________

Date	*Diet*	*Appetite*	*Instructions (Verbal)*	*Instructions (Written)*	*Patient Feedback*

Disposition: ______________________________

Continued dietary needs at discharge: ______________________________

____

____

Above needs communicated to: ______________________ on ______________.
(name) (date)

Signed ______________________________

Retain in inpatient record

Discharge Planning for Home Health Care
Copyright © 1994, Aspen Publishers, Inc.

Exhibit 7–16 Pastoral Care Screening Criteria

Patient name: ______________________________ Date: ______________

Room #: ______________________________

Living Arrangements	*Age*
____Alone	Over 65____
____Spouse	
____elderly, disabled	Over 75____
____working	
____home all day	Over 85____
____Extended family, specify ______________	
____Facility, specify ______________	Over 90____

Precare available after hospitalization?

Yes____ No____

Member organized church?

Yes____ No____ Specify ______________

Utilizes community resources?

Yes____ No____ Specify ______________

Pastoral care needed?

Yes____ No____

Counseling____ Ministerial____

Other, specify ______________

Posthospital planning ______________

Follow-up comments:

Seen by: ______________________________ Date: ______________

Original—retain in department files

DISCHARGE PLANNING FOR HOME HEALTH CARE
Copyright © 1994, Aspen Publishers, Inc.

◆ Chapter 8 ◆

External Linkages

COMMUNITY COLLABORATION AND NETWORKING

A prerequisite for any successful discharge planning/home care coordinator program is community networking. All individuals who contribute to the multidisciplinary discharge planning team of the hospital must be liaisons with their community-based counterparts and must be knowledgeable of the available resources within the community for posthospitalized patients. These individuals should be members and participate actively in their professional organizations and associations. These groups offer their participants an opportunity to share knowledge and to lend support to the needs of the group as a whole and are a resource to individual members. Professional groups contribute to the change process by efforts of their membership.

In possessing local and regional community resources, one of the primary informants could be the local United Way. Many United Way organizations have developed countywide guides for services within their service areas. A cross-index and listing of categories is provided based upon the needs most often encountered by individuals within the community. These guides provide various amounts of information ranging from a basic guide, which includes the telephone number and address of the provider, to a more comprehensive listing, which includes services, contact individuals, and operational hours.

A second source for human service resources often is found along with government resources in the blue pages of the telephone book or is available from local chambers of commerce.

Consultation of these basic areas begins developing your individual knowledge of available community resources. In addition, it is necessary to meet the people within your community's resources and to network further into the smaller, less visible support services and resources within any one community.

As the hospital discharge planner/home care coordinator becomes increasingly visible within the local community and develops one-to-one relationships with his or her community counterparts, the job of posthospital care and placement becomes easier. There develops a feeling of comradery, an understanding and appreciation of each other's constraints, and a willingness to help each other out when especially difficult posthospital care needs are apparent.

When available information is incomplete or nonexistent, the task of the discharge planner/home care coordinator is greater, and a planned community needs assessment is indicated. In Chapter 1, a community needs assessment outline was presented that focused on assessing the community need for better discharge planning by the hospital to develop a comprehensive hospital to home care discharge plan (see Exhibit 1–1). Our steps in this process remain the same, but our objective and focus in this needs assessment differ. It is often possible to combine these surveys into one survey tool that serves both purposes, but this becomes a more comprehensive project. For our purposes, we have chosen to complete these as separate surveys because often these needs are identified at separate times within the organization, or the organization has need of only one of the assessments.

The objective of this community needs assessment is to identify community resources available to assist patients and families after a hospitalization. The data-gathering sources identified in Exhibit 1–2 are similar sources for information, but the assessment format and actual survey tool differ.

In addition to the service providers identified as data-gathering sources in Exhibit 1–2, the following should be included in any community resource list:

- physical referral services
- nursing care services
- rehabilitation services
- clinical laboratories
- radiology service providers
- nutrition and weight loss services
- social service organizations
- transportation providers
- education/training providers
- financial assistance services
- pharmacies
- medical/adaptive equipment companies

- support groups
- legal aid services
- housing resources
- regulatory resources (such as Department of Environmental Resources)
- government resources
- employment agencies
- personal care/homemaker services
- home maintenance services
- health care providers
- fraternal organizations

An introductory letter such as that shown in Exhibit 8–1 should accompany a sample community survey tool (Exhibit 8–2). Once the data are obtained and summarized, the task force can distribute the report to interested participants and also utilize the data in discharge planning. If the health care organization is unwilling to undertake the funding for this project, the discharge planner should investigate alternative funding sources such as a health care grant, Office of Aging grant, state funds, or an individual benefactor within the community.

Besides utilizing the data obtained to meet the needs of patients being discharged from the hospital as well as the needs of the community at large, a survey also identifies gaps in services. Gaps can be evaluated for potential new program areas to be developed. Once this general community resource list is compiled, individual service components can be targeted for more indepth survey. In light of the Americans with Disabilities Act (ADA) of 1990 (see Appendix C), as a service for wheelchair-restricted citizens this task force could undertake a community needs assessment of community facilities that best meet the needs of mobility-restricted individuals. For example, all facilities could be assessed and recommendations made that would bring individual facilities into ADA compliance (Exhibit 8–3).

This task force, if it is a community-based task force, can be the initial point of networking for the health care provider's staff. As an offshoot of this task force's work, the participants should be able to identify the organizations and individuals within the community that could be of the most assistance in their roles as discharge planners/home care coordinators. This allows for the cost-effective use of their time in community liaison networking activities. Appendix D is a national resource list of health care service providers and a listing of human services organizations.

Exhibit 8–1 Introductory Letter to Accompany Community Survey Tool

Dear

On behalf of that segment of the population in need of supportive services within their homes, we at ABC Hospital have undertaken the task of assimilating a listing of the total resources available within our community.

We have formed a task force whose initial objective is the compilation of the findings from the attached survey. Because we recognize the need for input into our project from other human service providers, we invite you to participate in our task force.

If you are unable to become an active task force participant, we still request that you take a few moments to complete the attached survey and return it to us in the self-addressed stamped envelope by [date]. Please indicate on the survey whether your organization desires a copy of our report for utilization with your clients.

A prompt and complete response will assist us in the timely preparation of a valid resource tool for use by all of us in meeting our clients' needs.

Thank you for your time and interest in our project.

Sincerely yours,

Jane Doe
Community Resource Project Coordinator

DISCHARGE PLANNING FOR HOME HEALTH CARE
Copyright © 1994, Aspen Publishers, Inc.

Exhibit 8–2 Community Resource Survey

Correct Name of Agency: ______________________________

Address: ______________________________

____

Telephone number: ______________________________

Contact person: ______________________________

Title: ______________________________

Hours of operation: ______________________________

Information needed by agency: ______________________________

____

Services provided: ______________________________

____

____

Geographic area covered: ______________________________

____

____

Cost reimbursement sources: ______________________________

____

____

Sliding scale/uncompensated care protocols: Yes No

Specify: ______________________________

____

Volunteers utilized: Yes No

Task force interest: Yes No

Completed project requested: Yes No

____

____

Other comments: ______________________________

____

____

Completed by: ______________________________

Date: ______________________________

DISCHARGE PLANNING FOR HOME HEALTH CARE
Copyright © 1994, Aspen Publishers, Inc.

Exhibit 8–3 ADA Compliance Tool: Public Building Accessibility Evaluation (conforming to the American National Standards)

Name: ______________________________ Hours of operation: __________

Location: ______________________________ Phone: ______________

Services available: ______________________________

____

Contact person for special needs: ______________________________

Phone: ______________________________

I. Parking evaluation

_____Handicap area—Distance from building ___________feet to handicap area

___________feet to general parking

_____Drive-up facility

II. Building access

_____Curb ramps

_____maximum slope of 1″/12″

_____stable, firm, and slip-resistant surface

_____detectable warning texture

_____Ramp to access building

_____maximum slope of 1″/12″

_____stable, firm, and slip-resistant surface

_____minimum clear width of 36″

_____Doorway

_____minimum width of entrance 32″

_____two doors in a series—separation space of 48″ plus the width of any door

_____doors swing in the same direction or away from the space between the doors

III. Lavatory facilities

_____Entrance doors with minimum width of 32″

_____Unobstructed turning space/clear floor space (minimums vary with design, check local codes)

_____Sink height of 28″ to 32″ with 30″ clear floor space beneath

_____Grab bars in reinforced wall areas

DISCHARGE PLANNING FOR HOME HEALTH CARE
Copyright © 1994, Aspen Publishers, Inc.

THE CHANGE PROCESS

To facilitate the use of data gathered from community needs assessments conducted, it is often necessary to understand the change process. When any change takes place, there emerges someone as the facilitator for change. That person should be well versed in the background theories of change. Several well-known theorists and the major focus and impetus of their change theories are provided in Table 8–1. To become well versed in the theory most suited to the facilitator, it is recommended that individual research be conducted on these theories.

Perhaps one of the most well-known change theorists is Kurt Lewin. In 1947, Lewin propagated his theory of force field analysis of change. In this work, he described human behavior as being in a constant state of equilibrium with two forces at work against each other. These forces were identified as driving and restraining forces. Driving forces were further defined as forces pressuring movement toward something: the restraining forces resist that movement.

This describes the process of change within any given area. In the community or within any setting, once needs are assessed and there is a recognized need for change, forces are at work. The role of the facilitator or leader is to identify the driving forces and to strengthen these while working to reduce the restraining forces or to use a combination of these strategies. Weakening the restraining forces and increasing the power of the driving forces simultaneously once the change process is underway is one strategy further defined by Lewin's five-phase unfreezing–refreezing change theory (Table 8–2).

The process of change is rarely easy and often is slow, but with the use of the good problem-solving techniques identified in Chapter 2 combined with an understanding and practical application of the concept of change, new community resources can be developed. Needed changes within existing resources can then be brought about by the discharge planning team of the hospital.

Table 8–1 Theories of Change

Theorist	*Focus/Approach*	*Major Types of Impetus*
Lewin	Force Field	Restraining/Enabling
Leavitt	Approaches	Structural, technological, people
Bemes	Strategies	Rational, reeducative, coercive
Alson	Categories	Organizational dysfunction, expansion
Donnelly	Subsystems	Change technology, problem solving

Table 8–2 Lewin's Phases of Change

Phase 1: Unfreezing	*Phase 2: Problem/Diagnosis*	*Phase 3: Goal Setting*	*Phase 4: New Behavior*	*Phase 5: Refreezing*
Seen as time for readiness for action in areas of attitudes, maturation, behaviors	Seen as time to identify forces and influences, diagnose need, introduce change in most appropriate places	Seen as time for establishment of specific goals, setting direction for change, planning steps to accomplish change	Seen as time to experiment with new behaviors, reevaluate change and adjust	Seen as time for establishment of changes as permanent; assimilation into routine and areas of attitude, motivation, behavior
Readiness for change develops				Change is complete

◆ Chapter 9 ◆

The Effects of Reimbursement: Today and Tomorrow

Along with the advent of the regulation of health care reimbursement described in Table 9–1 come significant changes in the economic conditions of acute care facilities. Resource allocation decisions about the use of health care dollars emerged as the primary focus of third party reimbursement in the mid-1970s. Decisions about the spending of health care resource dollars were made in three primary areas: total amount of dollars available, cost effectiveness of the health care setting, and the method for provision of dollars for health care throughout the entire population.

The actual per capita health care cost increased by 830 percent in the years from 1965 to 1985. Of these health care dollars, approximately 60 percent were from private pay reimbursement sources, which included the insurance, self-pay, and other third party payor sectors. The remaining 40 percent of health care dollars were from public reimbursement sources and were divided between federal (approximately 30 percent) and state (approximately 10 percent) funding.

Managed care concepts emerged in the 1970s as the answer to rising health care costs. Providers of managed health care were paid on an annual capitation fee basis in exchange for the responsibility of providing all the individual's health care needs. Physicians and providers were a part of this system of care, and incentives were put in place to decrease the demands on the health care system.

Table 9–1 Comparison of Reimbursement Sources, 1991*

Reimbursement Source	*Description*	*Anticipated Patient Expense*
Health maintenance organization (HMO) and managed care plan	Managed care through own service providers Emphasis on preventive care Generic drugs Decreased duplication of services Prior authorization Packaged service contracts If guidelines above are met, pays total coverage with participating provider	Monthly premium Dollar amount per prescription Deductibles
Preferred provider organization (PPO)	Discontinuing with hospitals and physicians Copayments with use of outside service provider Prior authorization Package service contracts If guidelines are met, pays total coverage with participating provider	Monthly premium Dollar amount per prescription
Third party payor and 65-plus plan	Contractual arrangements established Covers $75.00 Medicare Part B and $676.00 Medicare Part A deductibles Covers 20% copay for Medicare	Monthly premium Noncovered services Unapproved amounts for nonparticipating providers
Medicare Part A, inpatient	First 60 days: Medicare pays based on diagnosis-related group (DRG), allowance 61–90 days } 91–150 days } Noncovered Beyond 150 days } Covers semiprivate room, special care areas, drugs, diet, lab tests, radiology, rehab services, etc.	$676.00 hospital admission Daily rate beyond $148.00 per day Daily rate beyond $296.00 per day None
Medicare Part A, skilled nursing facility	100% for first 20 days if skilled coverage certified by physician and admission follows a 3-day inpatient stay	Beyond rate of $74.00 per day for days 21 to 100 Balance ongoing

*subject to annual ongoing updates.

Table 9–1 continued

Reimbursement Source	*Description*	*Anticipated Patient Expense*
Medicare Part A, home health care	100% coverage for homebound, skilled care needs that are physician ordered	General household care needs Drugs, meals, blood
Medicare Part A, hospice	210 days of coverage if certified by a physician to be terminal and patient chooses hospice benefit; two 90-day periods and one 30-day period	5% for certain services to a maximum of $676.00 per year
Medical Part B, physicians	80% of approved amount after deductible is paid	$75.00 deductible 20% of approved amount
Medicare Part B, hospital outpatient services	80% of approved amount after deductible is paid	20% of approved amount
Medicare Part B, other: • ambulance • durable medical equipment • laboratory • outpatient therapy • prosthetic devices • radiology • radiation therapy	80% of approved amount after deductible is paid	20% of approved amount
Medicaid	Variable with each state	Variable with level of coverage

MANAGED CARE

The cost effectiveness of care priority led to the evolution of the managed care component of health care. Traditionally, HMOs and PPOs were the organizations associated with managed care, but this practice now extends to most third party payors. This process controls the extent of health care services provided to an individual, and the individual's care is usually directed by a case manager. Most often this case manager is a registered professional nurse, who determines when additional services are needed as well as the duration of these services.

Health care organizations that can comprehensively meet an individual's total health care needs from prehospitalization through postdischarge are best positioned to lead in capturing this health care market. Packaged proposals are being developed and marketed to the HMOs, PPOs, and third party insurers. These packages offer competitively priced one-stop shopping. Agreed upon reimbursement levels motivate the provider to actively seek to promote care in the least expensive medium. In light of these changes in reimbursement, it is certain that early discharge planning will continue to be a vital component of the health care arena of the 1990s and beyond the year 2000.

The first federally qualified HMOs became available to employers with more than 25 employees in 1973, when federal guidelines were established. Other efforts to decrease the rapidly increasing cost of health care included the 1981 decree that Medicaid population could be directed toward a limited number of Medicaid providers. This resulted in the bid and contract process that is now prevalent in many health care settings. Managed care enrollment of the Medicaid population has now increased to 12 percent, or more than 12 million of the medical assistance recipients.* Health care reform of the 1990s will have a major impact on individual coverage and reimbursement issues.

A second effort to decrease these costs was seen by the private health insurers' implementation of second opinions and preauthorization for service. Table 9–1 describes each of the most common reimbursement sources for health care.

For the Medicare recipient, it is necessary to determine whether the care provider has agreed to be a participating supplier of health care. When the health care provider agrees to become a participating provider, it means that the provider will accept as its total charge the Medicare-approved fee and that the individual is responsible for only 20 percent of the approved fee on the copay amount. This is paid by the individual or his or her supplemental private insurance policy. This is referred to as accepting an assignment on the bill for services.

COST EFFECTIVENESS OF CARE

Because of the implementation of the diagnosis-related group (DRG) mode of reimbursement for Medicare hospitalization, it has become increasingly important to decrease the length of stay and/or to find a more cost-effective method of care provision.

---

*DSH Medicaid Payments Frozen. *Hospitals* (20 December, 1992): 6.

Care management and managed care systems focus on the achievement of cost-effective, quality care and developing collaborative practice models to meet the needs of patients within specific time frames. These systems focus on early discharge planning. The streamlining of the care management systems has resulted in the emergence of the new terminology of clinical pathways.

The multidisciplinary process of implementing a clinical pathway establishes specific time sequences for standard outcomes to be achieved. These outcomes are expected to be achieved within the DRG-specific length of care. When more than one acute or chronic diagnosis exists, clinical pathways for these combined diagnoses are developed. Should the time frames not be met, there is a resulting increased use of the health care provider's resources (e.g., staff salaries and supplies), and variances are said to have occurred. These variances are then studied by the multidisciplinary team to determine their causes. Examples of causative factors can include practice tendencies, resource availability, and complicating factors in the patient's condition. Exhibit 9–1 is a sample format to be used in further development of the clinical pathway model. Early discharge is one of the primary focuses of the clinical pathway model and contributes to patient satisfaction and quality of patient care.

Home care's emergence is a cost-effective answer for provision of ongoing health care services. In addition to home care's cost effectiveness, hospitals have relied on home health care to meet the individual's needs in a familiar environment surrounded by familiar caregivers. Both these factors enhance the healing process and expedite recovery time. The nature of the home care service provision also allows for the development of trust and confidence in the caregiver because of the ongoing care provided by the same individual.

Home care schedules the patient's visits over a longer duration, thus allowing for self-care to be broken down into smaller, more manageable components. Additionally, this allows for skilled assessments and interventions throughout the posthospitalization care period, a time when complications most often arise.

LEGAL AND RISK MANAGEMENT PERSPECTIVE

Home care is often the care of choice from the standpoint of cost effectiveness, but it is also important in the legal and risk management perspectives. Hospitals are more vulnerable to the legal implications of their actions and are concerned that the individual being discharged from the acute care setting is returning to a safe environment. The hospital's risk manager should be involved when making difficult decisions as to appropriate, safe follow-up care.

The home care provider of today has become increasingly more skilled in the provision of highly technical care, such as central venous catheter care, care of ventilator-dependent patients, and the administration of chemotherapeutic agents within the home setting. It is important that the hospital discharge planner be confident of the capabilities and level of expertise of the staff within the community's home health agencies. The Joint Commission on Accreditation of Healthcare Organizations criteria and survey standards implemented in 1988 represent one comprehensive credentialing method of the home health agency's total

Exhibit 9–1 Format for the Development of Clinical Pathways

PATHWAY: ______________________________

Assigned Case Manager: ______________________________

		Admission			
	Preadmission	*Day 1*	*Day 2*	*Day 3*	*Day 4*
Testing					
Laboratory					
Radiology					
Cardiac					
Respiratory					
Other					
Preadmissions					
Consults					
Cardiac					
Specialty					
Inpatient					
Dietary					
Other					
Diet					
Treatments					
Medications					
Discharge planning					
Patient education					

DISCHARGE PLANNING FOR HOME HEALTH CARE
Copyright © 1994, Aspen Publishers, Inc.

Exhibit 9–1 continued

*Note: Mark all exceptions with an E and explain, sign, and date all entries

Exception	*Causative Factors*	*Action Plan*	*Results*

DISCHARGE PLANNING FOR HOME HEALTH CARE
Copyright © 1994, Aspen Publishers, Inc.

operation. Certification should indicate a high degree of competence on the part of the home health agency. Another similar credentialing method available to home health agencies is Community Health Accreditation Program (CHAP). Both credentialing bodies have obtained deemed status with federal/state survey standards which allows certification to be maintained as a result of a satisfactory survey.

If the patient believes that he or she is being discharged too soon from the acute care setting or that a noncoverage decision is not appropriate, he or she should request a review by a peer review organization (PRO) for a decision about the noncoverage and should provide input to the PRO as to the reasons for seeking reconsideration. The patient and his or her family need to be kept aware of the available remaining days of approved inpatient care so that they can plan appropriately.

In the 1991 health care cost containment regional report for south-central Pennsylvania, the average length of stay (ALOS) of the total inpatient population was down to 5.1 days. For the patient with pulmonary edema, this stay was 7.9 days; a patient admitted with heart failure had an ALOS of 8.1 days. The ALOS figures for the total Mid-Atlantic area during this time period was 10.12 days. A hospital with an organized discharge plan had an ALOS of 6.9 days.* The cost savings to a hospital are self-evident.

TOMORROW: AMBULATORY PATIENT GROUPS

One of the newest proposed revisions to the Medicare payment system is in the area of outpatient services. The Health Care Financing Administration (HCFA) had until September 1, 1991 to submit its recommendation for the full-scale reform of the outpatient payment system. The Prospective Payment Assessment Commission was designated as the group responsible to review the HCFA's recommendations and to make appropriate recommendations to Congress by March 1994.

In citing the need for reform in this area, the Prospective Payment Assessment Commission states that outpatient costs increased at an annual rate of 16 percent per year from 1983 to 1989. Because outpatient payments are still based on costs, the belief is that there is not enough incentive to cut costs in this area. The new Ambulatory Patient Groups (APG) payment model will probably have the greatest impact on this health care arena. The proposed reimbursement model will affect inpatient discharge planning, and the overall APG reimbursement system will necessitate increased discharge planning intervention in the ambulatory care areas of the hospital, such as outpatient surgery, outpatient testing, primary care centers, and emergency department service areas.

---

*Stauffer, C. Hospital cost below average hire. *Lancaster New Era* (1991): B1-B2; Hawkes, J. Hospital cost below average. *Intelligence Journal* (1991): A1-A3.

◆ Chapter 10 ◆

Integration with Alternative Health Care Settings

OVERVIEW

In today's hurry-up world of acute care discharge planning, patients are often discharged from the hospital to another health care institutional setting. These settings have seen an increasing responsibility to plan for the next step in the patient's discharge planning. This step is the patient's discharge from the institution to their home or to a long-term placement setting.

This chapter is intended to assist institutions in adapting the discharge plan described in Chapter 2 to meet their unique discharge planning needs. No matter what the health care setting, research has shown a similarity of elements to be included in any discharge plan. Exhibit 10–1 lists these elements for incorporation into the plan.

Current health care settings have been included in this chapter, but as emerging care concepts are developed these setting adaptations will be included as updates to this chapter as appropriate. An example of one such care concept is the subacute care facility. This facility is designed as an interim health care provider for patients such as the outpatient surgical patient in need of 24-hour postoperative support, hospice patients whose families require respite care, and patients whose highly technical needs are still apparent but whose stabilized condition eliminates the need for the acute care setting.

The postoperative patient and the technically dependent patient are two groups of patients in need of a formalized approach to discharge planning for themselves and their families. As

Exhibit 10–1 Common Elements of Discharge Plans

1. Definition and purpose
2. Institution's philosophy of discharge planning
3. Organizational structure
    - Responsibility and accountability
    - Role definition
    - Departmental networking
4. Objectives
5. Procedures for:
    - Casefinding
    - Assessment
    - Intervention/implementation
    - Resource utilization
    - Coordination of discharge planning
    - Documentation
    - Completion of discharge
6. Program evaluation

DISCHARGE PLANNING FOR HOME HEALTH CARE
Copyright © 1994, Aspen Publishers, Inc.

these facilities grow in number and as bed capacities increase, this area will have increased discharge planning needs.

For our purposes, we have included the following facilities for adaptation suggestions: skilled nursing/long-term care facilities, personal care homes, rehabilitation hospitals, Veterans Administration hospitals, and mental health facilities.

DISCHARGE PLANNING NEEDS OF A SKILLED NURSING/LONG-TERM CARE FACILITY

The skilled nursing facility is able to provide 20 days of full Medicare Part A coverage to patients with a continuing need for skilled care.

To qualify as a skilled nursing facility, there must be formal policies written under the advice of at least one physician, registered nurse, or medical staff member. A registered nurse must be on duty 24 hours a day, and at least one registered nurse must be a full-time employee of the facility. All patients are under the care of a physician, and clinical records are maintained.

The Discharge Planning Task Force for the skilled nursing facility could include the quality improvement utilization management specialist, the admissions/discharge planner, and

Table 10–1 Discharge Plan Task Force Members and Mission

Task	*Skilled Nursing Facility Members*	*Mission*
Task force implementation	Quality assurance/ quality improvement Utilization management Admissions Social work Therapist Nurses	Develop a comprehensive discharge plan that meets the needs of patients and families
Plan development and implementation	Quality assurance/ quality improvement Utilization management Admissions Social work Therapist Nurses	Identify barriers to discharge planning Identify strengths that exist to support discharge planning Establish communication flow patterns/protocols Identify types of admissions that are expected to be discharged from the facility Establish discharge planning screens Implement screens and discharge plan

Exhibit 10–2 Discharge Plan Components

Discharge Planning Team

- Admissions/discharge coordinator
- Nursing
- Therapy staff (occupational, physical, speech as available)
- Utilization management/quality improvement specialist
- Physician
- Dietitian

Community Resources

- Home health agencies
- Area agency of aging
- Personal care homes
- Outpatient services
- Day care
- Meals on Wheels

Screening Criteria

- Medicare/Medicaid
- Short-term placements
- Post–medical/surgical incident such as surgery, cerebrovascular accident, myocardial infarction, fractured hip

Discharge Planning Meetings

- Weekly on each short-term unit
- Bimonthly on long-term units

Meeting Format

- Unit nurse provides basic patient information
- Social worker/discharge planner identifies psychosocial components
- Therapists discuss prognosis
- Caregivers provide input on patient needs

DISCHARGE PLANNING FOR HOME HEALTH CARE
Copyright © 1994, Aspen Publishers, Inc.

nursing and therapy representatives. Restrictions might limit the committee's membership, but the tasks remain similar to those of any other setting (Table 10–1).

In many skilled nursing facilities, the task force and the implementation team members will be the same. For that reason, once the barriers to and strengths for discharge planning are identified, the members will develop the criteria and implement the discharge plan. If necessary, a social work or discharge planning consultant can be contracted on a per diem basis to coordinate the development of the discharge plan and procedures for the institution. The discharge plan components (Exhibit 10–2) have been provided for use in this process. A sample admission intake form (Exhibit 10–3) and a sample discharge referral form (Exhibit 10–4) have also been included.

Because physician availability is often limited in this setting, it is a good idea to determine what the physician's expectations for discharge might be at the time of the patient's admission to the facility, and ongoing communication channels should be established among the physician, the discharge planner, the patient, and the family. Discharge planning could be designated to the admission's counselor, the primary nurse, or the quality improvement/utilization management specialist. An individual who enthusiastically supports discharge planning is an ideal candidate for this responsibility.

DISCHARGE PLANNING NEEDS OF REHABILITATION HOSPITALS

The rehabilitation hospital has emerged to meet the next level of care for functionally disabled individuals after discharge from the acute care hospital. To meet the criteria for admission to this facility, there must exist a need for medical as well as rehabilitative care.

The rehabilitation facility is usually the first choice for placement of the rehabilitation patient. One area of concern for these patients and their families is that often the distance from their home to the facility is long. Because of this concern for proximity, alternative care settings might be chosen, such as rehabilitative home care or outpatient therapy. Another care option for the patient admitted to the rehabilitation facility is for the patient to be discharged to an alternative care setting.

Ongoing reimbursement of rehabilitative care is closely linked to progress. For that reason, most rehabilitation facilities have clearly organized systems in place to communicate the progress being made by the individual and to plan for inpatient course and discharge.

If a formal discharge plan is not in effect, the plan in Chapter 2 with minor adaptations could be utilized to establish one within the rehabilitation facility. These minor adaptations would include designating the physiatrist, a medical physician specially trained in rehabilitative medicine, as the head of the discharge planning team.

The other key members of the multidisciplinary team are consistent with the acute care setting's multidisciplinary team. These include the physical therapist, occupational therapist, and speech therapist who work with the patient as well as the rehabilitation nurse and social worker. All individuals will have focused their studies on the needs of the rehabilitation patient.

Exhibit 10–3 Skilled Nursing Facility Admission Intake

I. Personal Data

Full Name of Applicant ______________________________

Last Middle First

Address ______________________________

______________________________ Phone ______________________________

Residence ______________________________ How long ______________________________

Date of birth ______________________________ Citizenship ______________________________

Age __________ Sex __________

Marital status (circle one)

S M Wid Div Sep Name of spouse ______________________________ Age ______

Address of spouse ______________________________

If deceased, give date of death ______________________________

Father's name ______________________________ Birthplace ______________

Mother's maiden name ______________________________ Birthplace ______________

Religious affiliation ______________________________

Name of church ______________________________ Pastor ______________________________

Education ______________________________ Usual occupation ______________________________
(even if retired)

Name of physician ______________________________ Address

Living will ____Yes ____No ____Copy on record ____Code status

II. Financial Data

Social Security # ______________________________ Amount ______________

Medicare # ______________________________ Check ____A ____B

Other coverage ______________________________

Name and address of bank ______________________________

Savings/checking accounts ____Yes ____No

Approximate balance ______________________________

Certificates of deposit ______________________________ Bank ______________________________

Approximate amount ______________________________ Due date ______________________________

DISCHARGE PLANNING FOR HOME HEALTH CARE
Copyright © 1994, Aspen Publishers, Inc.

Exhibit 10–3 continued

Safety deposit box ______________________________

Will ______________________ Executor ______________________

Stocks and bonds _____Yes _____No Approximate amount ______________

Cash on hand _____Yes _____No Approximate amount ______________

Pensions received—Amount______________ Source ______________

Is Applicant a veteran?_____________ Dates of service ______________

Is there any real estate owned? ______________________________

Assessed value $______________ Real value $______________

Mortgages, etc. $ ______________________________

Is there any life insurance? ______________________________

If so, please list:

Policy #______________Value______________Company ______________

Policy #______________Value______________Company ______________

Policy #______________Value______________Company ______________

III. Family/Guardianship

Is there a legally appointed guardian? _____Yes _____No If yes, identify.

Name ______________________ Address ______________________

Telephone ______________________________

If no, emergency notification

Name ______________________ Address ______________________

Telephone ______________________________

Is there a durable medical power of attorney for health?

_____Yes, specify ______________________________

_____No

Child(ren)

Name(s)	Address	Telephone	Birth date

Discharge Planning for Home Health Care
Copyright © 1994, Aspen Publishers, Inc.

Exhibit 10–3 continued

Sibling(s)

Name(s)	Address	Telephone	Birth date

IV. Funeral Arrangements

Release property to:

Name ______________________________

Address ______________________________

Telephone number ______________________________

Funeral director:

Name ______________________________

Address ______________________________

Telephone Number ______________________________

Arrangements made _____Yes _____No

Financial sources:

Signature ______________________________ Date ____________________

Copy 1—patient chart

DISCHARGE PLANNING FOR HOME HEALTH CARE
Copyright © 1994, Aspen Publishers, Inc.

Exhibit 10–4 Skilled Nursing Facility Discharge Referral Form

Name ______________________________ Telephone number ____________

Address ____

Marital Status: S M W D

Place of residence prior to admission

____

Community resources utilized prior to admission

_____Home health _____Chore

_____Skilled _____Attendant care

_____Personal care _____Meals on Wheels

_____Office of Aging _____Support groups

Anticipated discharge needs

_____Nursing

_____Therapy

_____Equipment, specify

_____Activities of daily living, specify

_____Transportation

_____Support groups

_____Other

Discharge placement of patient choice ______________________________

Realistic? _____Yes _____No If no, specify alternative placement plan ____________________

____

Name ______________________________ Date ____________________

Copy 1—patient chart
Copy 2—department files

Discharge Planning for Home Health Care
Copyright © 1994, Aspen Publishers, Inc.

One process for discharge planning would be for all disciplines to implement complete intake assessments at the time of admission. The physiatrist would complete a review of the physical status of the patient, and the social worker would complete a psychosocioeconomic screen of the patient and family.

After these evaluations are completed, an initial intake conference is held with the multidisciplinary team members, the patient, and his or her family or significant other. At this conference, each contributor should outline long- and short-range goals for the patient with an expected date of achievement and maximum potential. Each discipline area lists three activity goals on a combined intake status projection summary (Exhibit 10–5) that focuses the direction of the treatment plan.

At the initial intake assessment, target dates for reassessment conferences are established based upon the goals and projected achievement dates established during the initial intake conference. Ongoing reassessment conferences maintain a focus on the forthcoming discharge of the patient. The social worker is able to coordinate community referrals for the support needed after discharge.

Historically, the discharge planning coordinator within most rehabilitation facilities has been the medical social worker because he or she serves as a liaison between the facility and the community resources.

Rehabilitation facility discharges have also been occurring more rapidly than in the past, and for that reason it is essential that a formal plan exist that contains specific time frames for completion of the intake assessments and initial intake conference. This conference should be conducted within 2 days of admission to the facility. To meet this criterion, it is necessary either to limit Friday and weekend admissions or to provide staffing of all program areas 7 days a week. Because of the budgetary implications of this decision, the plan requires administrative support so that there exists administrative backing for the established protocols.

DISCHARGE PLANNING NEEDS OF VETERANS ADMINISTRATION FACILITIES

Because Veterans hospitals provide a full spectrum of acute care services along with a full complement of staff, the discharge plan for these facilities would be similar to that outlined in the preceding chapters. The major difference in this health care setting is the impact of the government and military regulations on the standard operating procedures established. A second major difference is the requirements for form completion.

When an individual interfaces with the Veterans benefit system, specific application forms and medical certificates must be utilized. The Veterans Administration form 10-10 initiated in 1979 has had subsequent versions but is still in use for the veteran to apply for medical benefits. This form must be completed and processed before Veterans benefits can be received for hospital treatment, domiciliary care, outpatient medical/surgical services, outpatient dental care, and nursing home care. Additionally, the Veterans Administration forms 10-10m (medical certificate), 10-10f (financial work sheet), and 21-2680 (housebound status in permanent need of regular aide and attendant care) must be completed.

Exhibit 10–5 Intake Status Projection Summary

Name ______________________________

Address ______________________________

Telephone number ______________________________

Significant other ______________________________

Date of birth ______________ Social Security # ______________

Insurance 1) ______________________________

2) ______________________________

3) ______________________________

Diagnosis ______________________________

Marital status: M S W D

Date/ Initials	*Discipline*	*Activity/Focus*	*Goal*	*Projected Date of Achievement*
	Nursing	1.		
		2.		
		3.		
	Physical therapy	1.		
		2.		
		3.		
	Occupational therapy	1.		
		2.		
		3.		
	Speech therapy	1.		
		2.		
		3.		
	Social work	1.		
		2.		
		3.		

DISCHARGE PLANNING FOR HOME HEALTH CARE
Copyright © 1994, Aspen Publishers, Inc.

Exhibit 10–5 continued

Date/ Initials	*Discipline*	*Activity/Focus*	*Goal*	*Projected Date of Achievement*
	Dietary	1.		
		2.		
		3.		
	Patient	1.		
		2.		
		3.		
	Family	1.		
		2.		
		3.		
	Other	1.		
		2.		
		3.		

Follow-up Conferences

Date	*Discipline*	*Goal Revised*	*Status Update*

Discharge Planning for Home Health Care
Copyright © 1994, Aspen Publishers, Inc.

Exhibit 10–5 continued

Anticipated Discharge Plans

Date	*Location*	*Support Needed*

Copy 1—patient chart

Discharge Planning for Home Health Care
Copyright © 1994, Aspen Publishers, Inc.

Once these forms are completed and the veteran has been cleared for services, services must be preauthorized for provision through providers outside the Veterans Administration's health care system where Veterans Administration health care providers are not available.

The overcrowding in the Veterans Administration facilities in recent years has necessitated an increased emphasis on the discharge planning process. The discharge planner for the Veterans Administration hospital deals with veterans from a wide geographic area and for that reason needs sharpened expertise to identify the community resources available in different locales. The national resource list included in Appendix D should prove to be of value in the pursuit of that knowledge. It is recommended that a community resource profile form (Exhibit 10–6) be developed for major referral populations. This expedites the discharge process and facilitates the transition of the veteran to his or her home community.

DISCHARGE PLANNING NEEDS FOR PERSONAL CARE HOMES

Admissions to personal care homes are usually for individuals who are able to care for themselves but have a need for some supportive services, such as meal preparation, house cleaning, safety in transfers, or ambulation. In some instances where a skilled care need exists, the home health agency is able to send in a nurse or therapist to provide the skilled care under the direction of the physician and paid for by the recipient's Medicare or private insurance benefit. Once the skilled care required has stabilized or been completed, there is minimal physician involvement within this type of setting.

Personal care homes are utilized for some short-term placements, but in many cases the residents have chosen this lifestyle to meet their care needs on a long-term basis. Discharge planning within this setting therefore requires an ongoing assessment of the resident's ability to care for himself or herself. As signs of deterioration begin to occur, the discharge planning team, usually the owner or manager and the health care professional available on a daily basis, should undertake the completion of a resident inventory (Exhibit 10–7) to determine the appropriateness of the patient remaining in the personal care home.

At the time of admission, a resident preference inventory (Exhibit 10–8) of locations that meet the patient's future needs and financial capabilities should be completed. The resident preference inventory should be completed annually until signs of increasing dependence occur, at which time it is suggested that this form be reviewed on a 60-day basis so that the resident has been prepared for alternative placement if it becomes necessary. The resident preference inventory should also be updated annually, which will allow the information to be current and also valid when the need for other care arrangements arises.

DISCHARGE PLANNING NEEDS OF MENTAL HEALTH CARE FACILITIES

The recent evolution of mental health care has seen a decrease in lifetime and long-term admissions to facilities and an increase in short-term admissions. Acute behavioral and

Exhibit 10–6 Community Resource Profile

State ______________________________

Geographic area ______________________________

Major city(ies) ______________________________

Service Need/Type	*Provider*	*Address*	*Telephone*	*Contact Person*
Nursing home				
Home care				
Skilled				
Personal				
Outpatient therapy				
Dietary support				
Diagnosis support				
Closest Veterans Administration facility				

Date of profile ______________________________

Completed by ______________________________

Copy 1—department/administrative files

Discharge Planning for Home Health Care
Copyright © 1994, Aspen Publishers, Inc.

mental symptom exacerbations are frequently handled in outpatient or community-based treatment programs. These changes have meant that discharge planning has taken on a new emphasis within the mental health care provider arena, and an organized approach to the evaluation of the discharge potential for all patients must be completed.

Key members of this discharge planning team include the psychiatrist, psychiatric social worker, counselor, group therapy leader, musical and recreational therapist, and the nurse and unit caregivers. All these individuals have the opportunity to view the patient in a variety of structured and unstructured settings and can contribute to the postacute care plan for the patient.

The discharge plan outlined in Chapter 2 can easily be adapted to meet the discharge planning needs of the mental health facility. This plan will incorporate the key team members.

A sample intake assessment (Exhibit 10–9) has been included for use. This tool can be enlarged with the detail needed for the individual mental health facility. A mental health discharge planning work sheet (Exhibit 10–10) can also be utilized in planning for the post-acute care needs of the mental health patient. The postacute care needs mirror the medical/surgical patient's needs except for the increased emphasis on psychosocial support and community resources.

These are two sample tools to be utilized in the development of the total mental health discharge plan. Each individual discharge team member should identify the key components of discharge as it relates to his or her discipline and should either adapt the tool in Chapter 7 or develop one unique to his or her discipline utilizing these as baseline tools.

Discharge planning is increasingly important in mental health facilities because of the shrinking dollars available to provide mental health treatment. By earlier discharge and increased use of outpatient and community treatment, these dollars can be spread over a longer period of time and utilized more effectively.

Exhibit 10–7 Personal Care Resident Inventory

Name ______________________________

Admission date ______________ Diagnosis ______________

Functional level:
1. Independent
2. Assistance (minimal)
3. Moderate assistance needed
4. Dependent

Date	*Level*	*Item*	*Date*	*Level*	*Item*
______	______	Feeding/eating	______	______	Mental status (circle)
______	______	Food preparation	______	______	• Confused
______	______	Dressing	______	______	• Noisy
______	______	Bathing	______	______	• Combative
______	______	Shower/tub	______	______	• Withdrawn
______	______	Toileting			
______	______	Urine	______	______	Housekeeping (circle)
______	______	Bowels	______	______	• Laundry
______	______	Mobility	______	______	• Bed
______	______	Cane	______	______	• Room
______	______	Crutches			
______	______	Walker			
______	______	Wheelchair			
______	______	Vision			
______	______	Glasses Y/N			
______	______	Hearing aid Y/N			
______	______	Speech clear Y/N			
______	______	Medications			

Discharge Planning for Home Health Care
Copyright © 1994, Aspen Publishers, Inc.

Exhibit 10–7 continued

Date	*Suggestions To Assist with Independence*

Able to continue to meet criteria Y N

Comments: ______________________________

Alternative care sought Y N

Comments: ______________________________

1. Completed by ______________________________ Date ______________
2. Reviewed by ______________________________ Date ______________
3. Reviewed by ______________________________ Date ______________
4. Reviewed by ______________________________ Date ______________
5. Reviewed by ______________________________ Date ______________
6. Reviewed by ______________________________ Date ______________
7. Reviewed by ______________________________ Date ______________
8. Reviewed by ______________________________ Date ______________
9. Reviewed by ______________________________ Date ______________
10. Reviewed by ______________________________ Date ______________
11. Reviewed by ______________________________ Date ______________
12. Reviewed by ______________________________ Date ______________

Copy 1—on chart

DISCHARGE PLANNING FOR HOME HEALTH CARE
Copyright © 1994, Aspen Publishers, Inc.

Exhibit 10–8 Resident Preference Inventory

I, ______________________________, understand that at some point I may no longer meet the criteria necessary for remaining at ______________________________. At that time I would prefer the following postresidency care based upon availability and finances:

_____private nursing home, such as (in order of preference):

____

____

____

_____county nursing home

_____Veterans hospital

_____family care provided by (relative name and address in order of preference):

____

____

____

_____other, specify ______________________________

(Number the above from 1 to 5 in order of preference)

Signed ______________________________ Reviewed: ____________________
Resident

Date____________________

Date____________________

Date ______________________________ Date____________________

Witness ______________________________ Date____________________

Copy 1—file on chart
Copy 2—resident

Discharge Planning for Home Health Care
Copyright © 1994, Aspen Publishers, Inc.

Exhibit 10–9 Intake Assessment Checklist

Patient Name ____________________

Location ____________________

Admission date ____________________ Assessment date ____________________

Admitting physician ____________________

Primary diagnosis ____________________

Last admission ____________________

Third party payors

____Medicaid # ____________________

____Medicare # ____________________

____Veterans # ____________________

____CHAMPUS # ____________________

____Private Ins 1 ____________________

2 ____________________

____Self-pay

____Other

Assessment needs

____admitted for long-term placement

____return home evaluation

____evaluate support

____counseling evaluation

____psychosocial evaluation

____evaluate financial resources

____mental status evaluated

____confused ____oriented

____combative ____withdrawn

specify ____________________

DISCHARGE PLANNING FOR HOME HEALTH CARE
Copyright © 1994, Aspen Publishers, Inc.

Exhibit 10–9 continued

_____evaluate medical needs

_____diet _____skin

_____meds _____teaching

_____therapies, specify

_____PT _____OT _____ST

_____other medical needs

____

_____other needs

____

Signature______________________________Date ______________

Copy 1—chart
Copy 2—medical evaluation team
Copy 3—psychological evaluation team

Discharge Planning for Home Health Care
Copyright © 1994, Aspen Publishers, Inc.

Exhibit 10–10 Mental Health Facility Discharge Planning Work Sheet

Name ____________________

Address ____________________

Telephone number ____________________ Age ____________

Medicaid insurance ______________ Second insurance ______________

Place of residence before placement/admission

_____home, alone

_____home with family/significant other

_____home of ____________________

_____group home

_____no known place of residence

_____other

Community resources used before placement/admission:

_____home care

_____home health

_____Veterans

_____Meals on Wheels

_____chore/OOA worker

_____outpatient mental health services

_____identify ____________________

____

____

_____support group(s)

identify ____________________

____

_____AA

_____PA

_____Alanon

_____other

DISCHARGE PLANNING FOR HOME HEALTH CARE
Copyright © 1994, Aspen Publishers, Inc.

Exhibit 10–10 continued

Anticipated needs

_____nursing

_____physician

_____psychiatrist

_____therapist

_____counselor

_____group support

identify ______________________________

Activity needs

_____meals, special diet

____

_____personal care

_____medications

_____other, specify

_____house cleaning

_____transportation

_____finances

Other ____

Is return home realistic? _____Yes _____No

Signature ____ Date ______________________

Copy 1—patient file

DISCHARGE PLANNING FOR HOME HEALTH CARE
Copyright © 1994, Aspen Publishers, Inc.

◆ Chapter 11 ◆

Conclusion

THE OUTSIDE PROVIDER ROLE

The preceding chapters indicate that patient placement through the continuum of care doesn't occur without forethought, planning, organization, and commitment. Central to the process is the patient's interest. As an outside provider, it is sometimes difficult or confusing to determine who does what. It is our belief that the hospital needs to take a proactive approach with outside organizations, but failure to do so transfers the responsibility to the outside providers.

Some steps to enhance your working relationship are as follows:

- Contact the most appropriate discharge planning team member (the person with whom you interface the most) by phone to arrange a meeting; avoid appointments with multiple planning members to prevent misinterpretation of your intentions.
- Elicit information:
  1. What is the organization's discharge plan?
  2. Who is your liaison?
  3. When do you initiate contact?
  4. When can you expect to receive referrals?
  5. What format should you expect for referrals?

- Orient the liaison to your agency's operational mission, philosophy, and values:
  1. Does the liaison want your brochure?
  2. Does he or she know that you are your agency's liaison?
  3. Does he or she know the services you provide?
- Work within the organization's planning parameters.
- Develop positive relationships.
- Become certified by the Joint Commission on Accreditation of Healthcare Organizations, which will aid the organization's survey process in the area of quality of services.
- Maintain certification and state licensing credentials as applicable.
- Deliver the quality and quantity of service that are consistent with your marketing.
- Maintain professionalism with patient contacts.
- Support the organization in the social arena.
- Provide written feedback on postdischarge patient status (Exhibit 11–1).

TOTAL PLAN EVALUATION

Your institution's discharge plan should be reevaluated periodically to ensure that it is meeting the changing patient needs and community resources as reimbursement changes reshape the health care delivery system. Exhibit 11–2 can be adapted to individual facilities and offers guidelines for the evaluation process for use by the organization. This evaluation organization will enhance the effectiveness of the discharge plan.

"LET'S DO IT!"

This manual not only has emphasized the importance of discharge planning but also has provided a step-by-step approach to developing and implementing the plan. Like someone encountering a fork in the road, one could choose to veer off onto the path of complacency and refusal to change; after all, it is easier to avoid conflict by continuing to tolerate inertia. The other path, however, allows professionals within the institution to be accountable while utilizing their expertise in ensuring continuity of care for patients, who are the consumers of your service. A well-coordinated discharge plan is instrumental to your institution's success.

Exhibit 11–1 Agency Postdischarge Feedback

Dear______________________________,

Thank you for your assistance in the transfer of care from your hospital to our agency.

Mr./Mrs./Ms ____ was:

_____Admitted for services as planned on ______________________________.
(Date)

Currently, the patient's status is: ____

____

____

____

_____Admitted with changes in care as planned on ______________________________
(Date)

_____Not admitted as planned

Comment: ____

____

____

Sincerely,

____

Agency A Case Manager

DISCHARGE PLANNING FOR HOME HEALTH CARE
Copyright © 1994, Aspen Publishers, Inc.

Take This Test:

1. Do you want to support ongoing quality of care to your current customers?
2. Do you want your institution to provide reimbursable care?
3. Do you believe that a shorter length of stay will enhance your reimbursement?
4. Do you want to meet federal and state regulations?
5. Do you want to ease patient/family fears and insecurities with the organized use of your current staff?
6. Do you want to decrease acute care readmission rates?
7. Do you want to decrease posthospital complications?
8. Do you want to enhance your public image as the institution that cares about its patients as people?
9. As a community agency/facility, do you want to increase your referral base?

If you answered yes to four or more of these questions, then you have taken the first step toward effective discharge planning. You have identified the importance of the need.

Probably there are others in your organization who are in agreement. Informal internal networking will elicit supportive counterparts to begin your task force. The only way to get anything done is to begin. So let's do it!

Exhibit 11–2 Evaluation of the Discharge Plan

Mechanisms for Evaluation

- Patient satisfaction surveys
- Community agency/facility questionnaire feedback
- Multidepartmental discharge planning quality assurance/quality improvement reports
- Institutional length of stay statistics/financial status

Areas of Evaluation

1. Patient
   - Was the patient/family pleased with discharge planning procedures while in the hospital?
   - Were arranged services initiated as planned?
   - Were there consistently unidentified or unmet needs?
   - Does the patient have any suggestions to improve the planning process?
   - Was the patient pleased with the quality and quantity of follow-up services?
2. Community agencies/facilities
   - Were the referrals accurate and complete?
   - Were there needs that had not been identified?
   - Were follow-up phone calls/questions answered in a prompt and courteous manner?
   - Does the agency/facility have any suggestions to improve the planning process?
3. Multidisciplinary team members/departments
   - Do you have the opportunity to offer input into the discharge planning of the patient?
   - Is your input utilized in the planning process?
   - Are your verbal and written referrals complete and accurate? (If not, please explain)
   - Are your discharge planning tools functional and effective?
   - Do you have any suggestions to improve the organization's discharge plan?
4. Administration
   - Is the average length of stay at or below comparable area hospital statistics?
   - Is the marketing department aware of the results of the satisfaction surveys and questionnaires?
   - Are you receiving positive comments from middle managers, patients, physicians, and staff regarding discharge planning?
   - Are there any unmet needs due to lack of services in your community? If yes, can your institution address those needs?
   - Do you have any suggestions to improve the organization's discharge plan?

DISCHARGE PLANNING FOR HOME HEALTH CARE
Copyright © 1994, Aspen Publishers, Inc.

INSERT

TAB

◆ Appendix A ◆

Abbreviations

1 — primary
2 — secondary
AA — Alcoholics Anonymous
AAA — Area Agency on Aging
AARP — American Association of Retired Persons
ABG — Arterial blood gas
ADA — American Diabetes Association
ADA — Americans with Disabilities Act
ADL — Activities of daily living
Adm. — Admission
ALOS — Average length of stay
AHA — American Hospital Association
AHA — American Heart Association
APG — Ambulatory patient group
Appt. — Appointment
B.M. — Bowel movement
CCM — Clinical Case Manager
CD — Certificate of deposit
CHAP — Community Health Accreditation Program
CHF — Congestive heart failure
Coord. — Coordinator
COPD — Chronic obstructive pulmonary disease
COTA — Certified Occupational Therapy Assistant
CTA — Clear to ausculation
CVA — Cerebrovascular accident
CPR — cardiopulmonary resuscitation
D/C — Discharge
DER — Department of Environmental Resources
DDS — Doctor of Dental Surgery
DOE — Dyspnea upon exertion
DME — Durable medical equipment
DNR — Do not resuscitate
DO — Doctor of Osteopathy

DOA — Dead on arrival
DP — Discharge planning
DRG — Diagnosis-related group
DVR — Department of Vocational Rehabilitation
Dx — Diagnosis
ECF — Extended care facility
ECG — Electrocardiograph
EENT — Eye, ear, nose, throat
ESRD — End-stage renal disease
FBS — Fasting blood sugar
HCC — Home care coordinator
HCFA — Health Care Financing Administration
HHA — Home health aide
HHA — Home health agency
HHCC — Hospital health care council
HIV — Human immunodeficiency virus
HME — Home medical equipment
HMK — Homemaker
HMK/HHA — Homemaker/home health aide
HMO — Health maintenance organization
HOH — Hard of hearing
HSA — Health services administration
ICF — Intermediate care facility
i.m. — Intramuscular
IPR — Interpersonal relationship
IV — Intravenous
JCAHO — Joint Commission on Accreditation of Healthcare Organizations
JVD — Jugular vein distension
l — left
LLE — Left lower extremity
LOS — Length of stay
LPN — Licensed Practical Nurse
LTC — Long-term care
LUE — Left upper extremity
MA — Medical assistance
MC — Medicare
MD — Medical Doctor
MH — Mental health
MI — Myocardial infarction
MOW — Meals on Wheels
M/S — Medical/surgical
MSS — Medical social services
MSW — Medical Social Worker
NA — Nurse's aide
NBN — Newborn
O^2 — Oxygen
OB — Obstetrics
o.d. — Daily
OOA — Office of Aging
OT — Occupational Therapist
OVR — Office of Vocational Rehabilitation
PA — Physician's Assistant
PA — Parents Anonymous
PAT — Preadmission testing
PC — Personal care
PCC — Patient care coordinator
PCH — Personal care home
PD — Private duty
PEARL — Pupils equal and reactive to light
POA — Power of attorney
PPO — Preferred provider organization
PRO — Peer review organization
PROM — Passive range of motion
ProPAC — Prospective Payment Assessment Commission
PSRO — Professional Standards Review Organization
PT — Physical Therapist
Pt. — Patient
q — Every
QA — Quality assurance
QI — Quality improvement
r — Right
RBRVS — Resource-based relative value scale

RLE —Right lower extremity
RN —Registered Nurse
RT —Respiratory Therapist
RUE —Right upper extremity
Rx —Treatment
SASH —Saline, antibiotic, saline, heparinized saline
SE —Side effects
SHCC —State health coordinating council
SHPDA—State health planning and development agency
SNF —Skilled nursing facility
s.q. —Subcutaneous
SS —Social Security
SSA —Social Security Administration
ST —Speech Therapist
TBA —To be admitted
U —Units
UM —Utilization management
UR —Utilization review
VA —Veterans Administration
v.s. —Vital signs
WNL —Within normal limits
X —Times

◆ Appendix B ◆

Policies and Procedures

Policy number: 1

Subject: Discharge planning—Patient screening criteria

Policy: It is the policy of XYZ Healthcare to provide discharge planning services for all patients.

Procedure:

1. The standard of care for all patients includes identification of postdischarge needs by every professional providing direct care.
2. Timeliness of referrals to the social worker or home care coordinator is especially important for the following needs:
   - psychosocial status
     —older than 65
     —lives alone
     —lack of residence
     —lack of financial resources
     —lack of support

DISCHARGE PLANNING FOR HOME HEALTH CARE
Copyright © 1994, Aspen Publishers, Inc.

—poor cognition/altered mentation
—suspected abuse or neglect
—history of noncompliance
—admitted from skilled nursing facility, intensive care facility, or personal care home

- medical status
  —chronic illness
  —frequent readmissions to acute care
  —altered body image (e.g., colostomy, amputation)
  —open/draining skin condition
  —terminal illness
  —limited mobility secondary to fractures, trauma, cerebrovascular accident
  —necessity for subcutaneous, intramuscular, or intravenous medication
  —multiple complications
  —extensive surgery
  —need for long-term ventilator or oxygen support
  —new mother desiring adoption
  —inability for independent activities of daily living
  —new medication regime
  —inability to communicate

3. Inpatient units will screen every patient in a formalized patient discharge planning meeting at least weekly.
4. Ambulatory care areas will screen every patient at the time of the encounter.

DISCHARGE PLANNING FOR HOME HEALTH CARE
Copyright © 1994, Aspen Publishers, Inc.

Policy number: 2

Subject: Uncompensated care

Policy: In accordance with the mission and philosophy of XYZ Healthcare, it is the policy to provide uncompensated care to the active, needy patient with inadequate financial resources who is part of the health care system.

Procedure:

1. Uninsured/underinsured patients are referred to the social worker for financial planning.
2. State and/or federal financial assistance applications are completed by the patient with the help of the social worker when appropriate.
3. The uncompensated care application is completed by the patient with the help of the social worker when no other source of funding is available (see Exhibit B–1).
4. The completed uncompensated care application is forwarded to the patient accounts division of the finance department.
5. A patient accounts financial representative reviews the information and provides written notification to the patient within 2 weeks (see Exhibit B–2).
6. Uncompensated care amounts are summarized by the patient accounts division of the finance department for inclusion in the hospital's cost report.

Copyright © 1994, Aspen Publishers, Inc.

Exhibit B–1 Uncompensated Care Application

Patient name ______________________________

Address ______________________________

____

Phone number ______________________ Do you: ____ own

____ rent

____ other

Explain ______________

____

____

Next of kin name ______________________________

Address ______________________________

____

Phone number ______________________________

Employment status: ____ unemployed ____ employed

Employer name ______________________________

Address ______________________________

____

Type of work ______________________________

How long ______________________________

Family size ______________________________

Financial assets

Salary	________	/month
Public assistance	________	/month
Disability	________	/month
Pension	________	/month
Rent	________	/month
Savings balance	________	
Checking balance	________	
Other bank holdings (CDs, money markets, etc.)	________	

DISCHARGE PLANNING FOR HOME HEALTH CARE
Copyright © 1994, Aspen Publishers, Inc.

Exhibit B–1 continued

Additional/family income ______________

TOTAL [ ]

Financial liabilities

Rent/mortgage ______________ /month

Prescription costs (include recent receipt) ______________ /month

Outstanding medical bills ______________

Other (explain): ______________________________ ______________

______________________________ ______________

______________________________ ______________

TOTAL [ ]

Health care needs by XYZ Healthcare (include type of care and dates) ______________________________

____

____

____

My signature indicates that the above information is accurate and correct to the best of my knowledge. I am aware that completion of this application does not necessarily indicate agreement by XYZ Healthcare to provide uncompensated care. I am aware that a financial representative will notify me in writing within 2 weeks of receipt of this application with information regarding the outcome.

Patient signature ______________________________ Date ______________

Copyright © 1994, Aspen Publishers, Inc.

Exhibit B–2 XYZ Healthcare

Date______________

Dear______________________________________,
Patient

Your application for uncompensated care has been reviewed by the Patient Accounts Division of the Finance Department. We have determined that:

_____ you do not qualify for uncompensated care.

_____ you qualify for a rate reduction of _________ percent for care provided from __[date]__ to __[date]__.

_____ you do not qualify for a rate reduction but do qualify for a prolonged payment schedule of $_________/month × _________ months.

Should you have any questions, please call me between 1 P.M. and 3 P.M. Monday through Thursday at ___phone number___.

Sincerely,

Representative Name
Financial Representative

DISCHARGE PLANNING FOR HOME HEALTH CARE
Copyright © 1994, Aspen Publishers, Inc.

Policy number: 3

Subject: Interdepartmental collaboration

Policy: It is the policy of XYZ Healthcare's multidisciplinary discharge planning team to collaborate throughout the planning process.

Procedure:

1. All discharge planning activities are written in the progress note section of the patient record. For ambulatory care patients with only single page records, the progress note is utilized and permanently affixed.
2. In addition to the above, it is the responsibility of each team member to communicate verbally when time constraints exist.
3. As each discipline finalizes its portion of the discharge plan, it must record onto the Interdepartmental Collaboration Record (see Exhibit B–3) for information purposes. This accurate information can be transferred onto the final patient discharge instruction sheet.
4. The Interdepartmental Collaboration Record is a permanent part of the record.

Discharge Planning for Home Health Care
Copyright © 1994, Aspen Publishers, Inc.

Exhibit B–3 Interdepartmental Collaboration Record, Final Discharge Plan

Disposition
______ Home—no follow-up services
______ Home—supportive services
______ SNF ______
______ ICF ______
______ PCH ______
______ Other ______

Equipment/supplies

Type	*Coordinated by*	*Provider of Patient Choice*	*Date Ordered*

Services

Type	*Coordinated by*	*Provider of Patient Choice*	*Date Ordered*
Skilled home care			
__nursing			
__PT			
__OT			
__ST			
__MSS			
__aide			
Private Duty Care Level______ Hours			

Addressograph

DISCHARGE PLANNING FOR HOME HEALTH CARE
Copyright © 1994, Aspen Publishers, Inc.

Policy number: 4

Subject: Initiation of patient instructions

Policy: It is the policy of XYZ Healthcare to initiate anticipated patient instructions early in the hospitalization.

Procedures:

1. The standard of care for all patients includes identification of patient education needs by every professional providing direct care.
2. A special emphasis on timely initiation of patient education needs to occur with the following:
   - new medication regime
   - need for prosthetic device, including indwelling catheter
   - need for special procedures, such as:
     —respiratory treatments
     —ostomy appliance changes
     —wound care
     —injections
   - new diagnosis
3. The patient's status in the learning process will be conveyed to the postdischarge care provider by the coordinating discharge planning team member. The Patient Instruction Checklist (see Exhibit B–4) is to be utilized, with a copy going to the postdischarge provider.

Discharge Planning for Home Health Care
Copyright © 1994, Aspen Publishers, Inc.

Exhibit B–4 Patient Instruction Checklist (Date and Initial Each Entry)

Insulin-Dependent Diabetes Mellitus

Item	*Instruction/ Reinstruction*	*Patient Demonstration*
1. Disease process		
2. Signs of hypoglycemia		
3. Treatment of hypoglycemia		
4. Signs of hyperglycemia		
5. Treatment of hyperglycemia		
6. Use of oral hypoglycemic agents		
7. Types/use of insulin		
8. Storage of supplies		
9. Supply purchase, insulin administration		
10. Gathering supplies		
11. Handwashing		
12. Preparation of syringe		
13. Cleansing insulin vial		
14. Injection of air into vial		
15. Inversion of vial		
16. Aspiration of insulin into syringe		
17. Site selection		
18. Site rotation		
19. Cleansing of site		
20. Insulin injection		
21. Needle withdrawal		
22. Sharps disposal		

Date	*Initials*	*Signature*

Addressograph

DISCHARGE PLANNING FOR HOME HEALTH CARE
Copyright © 1994, Aspen Publishers, Inc.

Policy number: 5

Subject: Short-term skilled nursing facility placement follow-up

Policy: It is the policy of XYZ Healthcare to establish a multileveled discharge plan for the patient in need of temporary skilled nursing facility placement.

Procedure:

1. The social worker and home care coordinator will discuss posthospital options with the patient.
2. When necessary, a family meeting will be arranged to discuss options, financial responsibilities, and expected patient needs.
3. The social worker will provide the patient and family, if indicated, with the names of skilled nursing facilities for completion of order of preference.
4. The social worker will coordinate transfer needs while serving as a liaison between the skilled nursing facility and the hospital.
5. The home care coordinator will provide the patient and family, if indicated, with the names of home care providers for patient choice.
6. The home care agency of the patient's choice will be notified of the patient's temporary skilled nursing facility placement and projected need for skilled home care.
7. The home care agency will be responsible for following up with the skilled nursing facility.
8. The patient will be made aware of the status of the home care referral.

Discharge Planning for Home Health Care
Copyright © 1994, Aspen Publishers, Inc.

Policy number: 6

Subject: Postdischarge follow-up

Policy: It is the policy of XYZ Healthcare to contact the patient by phone within 48 hours of the discharge.*

Procedure:

1. The patient's primary nurse assumes responsibility for the postdischarge follow-up.
2. A copy of the patient's discharge instruction sheet is utilized in the process.
3. Newly identified problems are referred to the most appropriate member of the discharge planning team for follow-up.
4. Patients discharged to skilled nursing facilities do not receive a postdischarge follow-up call.

*Refer to Tables 6–2 and 6–3.

DISCHARGE PLANNING FOR HOME HEALTH CARE
Copyright © 1994, Aspen Publishers, Inc.

Policy number: 7

Subject: General administrative discharge plan policy

Policy: It is the policy of XYZ Healthcare to provide discharge planning to the patients in its care.

Procedure:

1. A comprehensive discharge plan will be established that will utilize the expertise of the institution's human resources.
2. The plan will be reviewed and revised at least annually.
3. The plan will be forwarded to department directors encompassing the multidisciplinary team.

DISCHARGE PLANNING FOR HOME HEALTH CARE
Copyright © 1994, Aspen Publishers, Inc.

◆ Appendix C ◆

The Americans with Disabilities Act and Its Impact on Health Care Facilities

Contributed by Jade Ann Gingerich,
American Association of State Colleges and Universities,
Washington, DC, 1992

WHAT IS THE AMERICANS WITH DISABILITIES ACT?

The Americans with Disabilities Act (ADA), which was signed into law on July 26, 1990, is considered the single most important piece of civil rights legislation since the Civil Rights Bill of 1964. The ADA legislation was introduced to give recognition and legal recourse to the 43 million persons with disabilities. In spite of improvements after the passage of Section 504 of the Rehabilitation Act of 1973, persons with disabilities have continued to experience discrimination in such critical areas as employment, housing, public accommodations, education, transportation, communication, recreation, institutionalization, health services, voting, and access to public services.

For the many institutions that have been in compliance with Section 504, the passage of the ADA will not require them to make numerous modifications. The historical commitment of many health care facilities to go beyond the minimum requirements will be rewarded with the need to implement only minor changes to be in full compliance with the ADA. Certainly in some areas, facilities will find that even with the passage of the ADA they still enjoy a leadership role in meeting the needs of the persons with disabilities in their community.

Discharge Planning for Home Health Care
Aspen Publishers, Inc.

WHAT DOES THE AMERICANS WITH DISABILITIES REQUIRE?

The ADA requires that all private businesses, state and local governments, employment agencies, labor unions, and public entities provide access for persons with disabilities to public services, accommodations, and transportation. It prohibits discrimination in the hiring and promotion of qualified persons with disabilities and requires that interstate and intrastate telecommunications relay services be available to persons who are hearing and speech impaired.

WHAT IS A DISABILITY?

The Act, for its purposes, has defined a person with a disability as follows:

- an individual with a physical or mental impairment that substantially limits one or more major life activities
- an individual with a record of such an impairment (for example, a history of cancer)
- an individual who is regarded or treated as having a disability (for example, facial disfigurement) even though he or she may not have such an impairment.

WHAT ARE THE IMPORTANT DEADLINES?

The deadlines for compliance are as follows:

- Title I: employment—July 26, 1992
  Prohibits discrimination against persons with disabilities in all employment practices and all employment-related activities

- Title II: public services—January 26, 1993
  Prohibits exclusion of persons with disabilities from participation in, and prohibits such persons from being denied, the benefits of services, programs, or activities of a public entity

- Title III: public accommodations—January 26, 1993
  Prohibits discrimination on the basis of disability in the full and equal enjoyment of goods, services, facilities, privileges, advantages, or accommodations of any place of public accommodation

- Title IV: telecommunications—July 26, 1993
  Provides for the implementation of regulations for common carriers to establish and offer telecommunication services on an equivalent basis for the hearing and speech impaired.

The Act requires changes that are readily achievable without requiring undue hardship. *Readily achievable* is defined in the Act as meaning easily accomplishable and able to be carried out without much expense or difficulty. *Undue hardship* is specified as an action requiring significant difficulty or expense.

An employer is only required to accommodate a known disability.

HOW WILL THE AMERICANS WITH DISABILITIES ACT AFFECT HEALTH CARE FACILITIES?

Health care facilities will be responsible for ensuring that persons with disabilities have:

- physical access to buildings, grounds, and facilities and facility-sponsored transportation, when appropriate
- employment opportunities and advancement
- physical and cognitive access to clinical program areas and health education programs

The regulations of the ADA are complex and in many cases specific or on a case-by-case basis. Therefore, it is recommended that legal counsel be sought as institutions move to comply with the ADA. These guidelines are not intended to be a substitute for legal counsel.

WHERE CAN ADDITIONAL INFORMATION BE OBTAINED?

Copies of the ADA can be obtained from:

House Document Room
Room B 18
Annex 2
Washington, D.C. 20515
(202) 225-3456

Request Public Law 101-336. Only written requests will be honored. Include a self-addressed stamped envelope to expedite receipt of materials.

Guidelines on public services and public accommodations can be obtained from the Department of Justice [(202) 514-0301, (202) 514-0381 TDD]. Guidelines on employment requirements can be obtained from the Equal Employment Opportunity Commission [(202) 663-4900, (800) 800-3302 TDD; in Washington, D.C.: (800) 663-4494 TDD]. Guidelines on telecommunications issues can be obtained from the Federal Communications Division [(202) 632-7260, (202) 632-6999 TDD]. Guidelines on transportation requirements can be obtained from the Department of Transportation [(202) 366-9305, (202) 755-7687 TDD]. Guidelines regarding requirements for new construction and alterations can be obtained from the Architectural and Transportation Barriers Compliance Board [(202) 663-4900, (800) USA-ABLE, (800) USA-ABLE TDD]. There is no charge for copies of these documents.

For further information about disabilities issues, contact:

- The National Organization on Disabilities [(800) 248-2253]
- The Disability Rights Education and Defense Fund [(800) 466-4232]

◆ Appendix D ◆

National Resource List

Name	*Address/Phone*	*Brief Function Description*
ACTION	1100 Vermont Avenue N.W. Washington, DC 20525 (202) 634-9380	Volunteer programs
Administration on Aging	330 Independence Avenue S.W. Washington, DC 20201 (202) 245-0641	Federal government programs
Aging Network Services	Suite 907 4400 East-West Highway Bethesda, MD 20814 (301) 657-4329	For-profit social workers for case management
Alzheimer's Association	Suite 600 70 East Lake Street Chicago, IL 60601 (312) 853-3060	24-Hour hotline on Alzheimer's research and support

DISCHARGE PLANNING FOR HOME HEALTH CARE
Copyright © 1994, Aspen Publishers, Inc.

American Association of Homes for the Aging	Suite 400 1129 20th Street N.W. Washington, DC 20036-3489 (202) 296-5960	Professional organization of nonprofit nursing homes, other housing, and community service agencies
American Association of Retired Persons	1909 K Street N.W. Washington, DC 20049 (202) 872-4700	To improve quality of life for the older population
American Cancer Society	1599 Clifton Road N.E. Atlanta, GA 30329 (404) 320-3333 (800) 227-2345	Cancer research and education
American Council for the Blind	Suite 1100 1010 Vermont Avenue N.W. Washington, DC 20005 (202) 393-3666 (800) 424-8666	To improve living conditions of the visually impaired
American Diabetes Association	1660 Duke Street Alexandria, VA 22314 (703) 549-1500 (800) 232-3472	Diabetes research and education
American Dietetic Association	Suite 800 216 West Jackson Boulevard Chicago, IL 60606 (312) 899-0040	Professional dietitian association
American Federation for Aging Research	725 Park Avenue New York, NY 10021 (212) 570-2090	Research regarding the aging process
American Foundation for the Blind	15 West 16th Street New York, NY 10011 (212) 620-2147 (800) 232-5463	To assist the visually impaired to achieve independence

DISCHARGE PLANNING FOR HOME HEALTH CARE
Copyright © 1994, Aspen Publishers, Inc.

American Geriatrics Society	Suite 400 770 Lexington Avenue New York, NY 10021 (212) 308-1414	Professional organization of physicians and health care providers
American Health Care Association	1201 L Street N.W. Washington, DC 20005 (202) 842-4444	Represents the interests of health care facilities to Congress and federal regulatory groups
American Health Foundation	320 East 43rd Street New York, NY 10017 (212) 953-1900	Research in preventive medicine
American Heart Association	7320 Greenville Avenue Dallas, TX 75231 (214) 750-5397	Research and public education
American Hospital Association	840 North Lake Shore Drive Chicago, IL 60611 (312) 280-6000 (800) 242-2626	Represents hospitals and other health care facilities
American Lung Association	1740 Broadway New York, NY 10019-4374 (212) 315-8700	Education and research on lung disease
American Medical Association	535 North Dearborn Street Chicago, IL 60610 (312) 645-5000	Physician representation
American Nurses Association	2420 Pershing Road Kansas City, MO 64108 (816) 474-5720	Registered Nurse representation
American Occupational Therapists Association	P.O. Box 1725 1383 Picard Drive Rockville, MD 20850-4375 (301) 948-9626	Occupational Therapist representation

DISCHARGE PLANNING FOR HOME HEALTH CARE
Copyright © 1994, Aspen Publishers, Inc.

American Osteopathic Association	142 East Ontario Street Chicago, IL 60611 (312) 280-5857	Doctors of Osteopathy representation
American Parkinson's Disease Association	Suite 417 116 John Street New York, NY 10038 (212) 732-9550	Research and education regarding Parkinson's disease
American Physical Therapy Association	1111 Fairfax Street Alexandria, VA 22314 (703) 684-2782	Physical Therapist representation
American Red Cross	18th & D Streets N.W. Washington, DC 20006 (202) 737-8300	Health education, blood services, and disaster relief
American Society of Aging	Suite 572 833 Market Street San Francisco, CA 94103 (415) 543-2617	Quality of life issues of older persons
American Speech-Language-Hearing Association	10801 Rockville Pike Rockville, MD 20852 (301) 897-5700 (800) 638-8255	Research in communication disorders
Arthritis Foundation	1314 Spring Street N.W. Atlanta, GA 30309 (404) 872-7100	Research and education in arthritis
Better Vision Institute	Suite 1310 1800 North Kent Street Rosslyn, VA 22209 (703) 243-1528	Education in vision care
B'nai B'rith International	1640 Rhode Island Avenue N.W. Washington, DC 20036 (202) 857-6600	Assists those of Jewish faith

DISCHARGE PLANNING FOR HOME HEALTH CARE
Copyright © 1994, Aspen Publishers, Inc.

Catholic Charities	1319 F Street N.W. Washington, DC 20004 (202) 639-8400	Assist with a broad range of social needs
Children of Aging Parents	2761 Trenton Road Levittown, PA 19056 (215) 945-6900	Support to caregivers of older persons
Community Action Plan	(800) 732-0018 Check directory assistance for local office	Community issues
Disabled American Veterans	P.O. Box 14301 Cincinnati, OH 45250 (606) 441-7300	Represents veterans with service connected disabilities
Environmental Protection Agency	Public Information Center 401 M Street S.W. Washington, DC 20460 (800) 424-9346	Environmental Issues
Episcopal Society for Ministry on Aging	317 Wyandotte Street Bethlehem, PA 18015 (215) 868-5400	Support programs for older adults
Federal Council on Aging	Room 4280, HHS-N 330 Independence Avenue S.W. Washington, DC 20201 (202) 245-2451	Advisory group
Foundation for Hospice and Home Care	519 C Street N.E. Washington, DC 20002 (202) 547-7424	Professional and paraprofessional care for individuals at home
Health Care Financing Administration	200 Independence Avenue S.W. Washington, DC 20201 (800) 638-6833	Coordinates federal government in Medicare and Medicaid

Copyright © 1994, Aspen Publishers, Inc.

Health Insurance Association of America	Suite 1200 1025 Connecticut Avenue N.W. Washington, DC 20036 (202) 223-7780 (800) 423-8000	Information about health and disability insurance
Help for Incontinent People	P.O. Box 544 Union, SC 29379 (803) 579-7900	Patient advocacy and education
Huntington's Disease Society of America	6th Floor 140 West 22nd Street New York, NY 10011 (212) 242-1968 (800) 345-4372	Serves patients with Huntington's disease
Legal Services for the Elderly	3rd Floor 132 West 43rd Street New York, NY 10036 (212) 391-0120	Advisory center for legal problems of the elderly
Leukemia Society of America	733 Third Avenue New York, NY 10017 (212) 573-8484	Research on leukemia and blood-forming diseases
Link Up America	Initial contact to this number for information re: locality (800) 332-1124	Networking among agencies
Lupus Foundation of America	Suite 203 1717 Massachusetts Avenue N.W. Washington, DC 20036 (202) 328-4550 (800) 558-0121	Research and public education on systemic lupus erythematosus

Discharge Planning for Home Health Care
Copyright © 1994, Aspen Publishers, Inc.

National AIDS Information Clearinghouse	P.O. Box 6003 Rockville, MD 20850 (800) 458-5231 (publications) (800) 342-2437 (hotline) (800) 344-SIDA (Spanish hotline)	Public and professional education on AIDS
National Arthritis and Musculo-skeletal and Skin Diseases Information Clearinghouse	P.O. Box AMS Bethesda, MD 20892 (301) 468-3235	Up-to-date information about these diseases
National Association for Hispanic Elderly	Suite 270 2727 West South Street Los Angeles, CA 90057 (213) 487-1922	To ensure elderly Hispanics' inclusion in social service programs
National Association for Home Care	519 C Street N.E. Washington, DC 20002 (202) 547-7424	Represents home care organizations
National Association for the Deaf	814 Thayer Avenue Silver Spring, MD 20910 (301) 587-1788	Information about and advocacy for deafness
National Association of Area Agencies on Aging	Suite 208W 600 Maryland Avenue S.W. Washington, DC 20024 (202) 484-7520	Represents the more than 650 area agencies on aging
National Association of Community Health Centers	Suite 122 1330 New Hampshire Avenue N.W. Washington, DC 20036 (202) 659-8008	Represents local health programs that serve the medically needy

Discharge Planning for Home Health Care
Copyright © 1994, Aspen Publishers, Inc.

National Association of Meal Programs	204 E Street N.E. Washington, DC 20002 (202) 547-5360	Congregate and homebound delivered meals
National Association of Social Workers	750 1st Street N.E. Suite 700 Washington, DC 20002-4241 (202) 408-8600	Professional organization of social workers
National Association of State Units on Aging	Suite 304 2033 K Street N.W. Washington, DC 20006 (202) 785-0707	Information, technical assistance, and support to state units on aging
National Cancer Institute	Office of Cancer Communications Building 31, Room 10A24 9000 Rockville Pike Bethesda, MD 20892 (301) 496-5583 (800) 4-CANCER	Research and information about cancer
National Caucus and Center on Black Aged	Suite 500 1424 K Street N.W. Washington, DC 20005 (202) 637-8400	To improve quality of life for elderly African Americans
National Center for Health Statistics	3700 East-West Highway Hyattsville, MD 20782 (301) 436-8500	Collects, analyses, and distributes health care data
National Council of Senior Citizens	925 15th Street N.W. Washington, DC 20005 (202) 347-8800	Advocacy for older Americans
National Council on the Aging	West Wing 100 600 Maryland Avenue S.W. Washington, DC 20024 (202) 479-1200	National resource for aging research and training

DISCHARGE PLANNING FOR HOME HEALTH CARE
Copyright © 1994, Aspen Publishers, Inc.

National Diabetes Information Clearinghouse	Box NDIC Bethesda, MD 20892 (301) 468-2162	Information about diabetes
National Digestive Diseases Information Clearinghouse	Box NDDIC Bethesda, MD 20892 (301) 468-6344	Information about digestive disorders
National Eye Institute	Information Office Building 31, Room 6A29 Bethesda, MD 20892 (301) 496-5248	Funding for eye research and distribution of information about eye diseases
National Foundation for Long Term Care	Suite 402 1200 15th Street N.W. Washington, DC 20005 (202) 659-3148	Works on behalf of long-term care providers and the chronically ill
National Geriatric Institute	212 West Wisconsin Avenue Milwaukee, WI 53203 (414) 283-7300	To advance the quality of care of the elderly, chronically ill, and disabled
National Heart, Lung, and Blood Institute	Information Office Building 31, Room 4A21 9000 Rockville Pike Bethesda, MD 20892 (301) 496-4236	Research and information about diseases of the heart, lung, and blood
National High Blood Pressure Information Center	4733 Bethesda Avenue Bethesda, MD 20814 (301) 951-3260	Educational materials on high blood pressure
National Hispanic Council on Aging	2713 Ontario Road N.W. Washington, DC 20009 (202) 265-1288	To promote the well-being of older Hispanics
National Hospice Association	Suite 901 1901 North Moore Street Arlington, VA 22209 (703) 243-5900	To promote the quality of care for the terminally ill

Discharge Planning for Home Health Care
Copyright © 1994, Aspen Publishers, Inc.

National Indian Council on Aging	P.O. Box 2088 Albuquerque, NM 87103 (505) 242-9505	Ensures that older native Americans and Alaskan natives have equal access to health care and legal and social services
National Information Center on Deafness	Galludet University 800 Florida Avenue Washington, DC 20002 (202) 657-5051 (voice) (202) 657-5052 (TDD) (800) 672-6720	Information about deafness
National Institute on Aging	Public Information Office Federal Building, Room 6C12 9000 Rockville Pike Bethesda, MD 20892 (301) 496-1752	Conducts and supports research on special problems of the elderly
National Institute on Alcohol Abuse and Alcoholism	Room 16-95 5000 Fisher Lane Rockville, MD 20857 (301) 443-1677	To develop strategies to deal with health issues associated with alcohol abuse
National Institute on Allergy and Infectious Disease	Office of Communications Building 31, Room 7A32 9000 Rockville Pike Bethesda, MD 20892 (301) 496-5717	Research on allergic, immunologic, and infectious diseases
National Institute on Arthritis and Musculoskeletal Diseases	Information Office Building 31, Room B2B15 9000 Rockville Pike Bethesda, MD 20892 (301) 496-8188	Research on arthritis and musculoskeletal diseases
National Institute on Community Based Long Term Care	409 Third Street S.W. Washington, DC 20024 (202) 479-1200 (202) 479-0735 (fax)	Support to community-based long-term care providers

DISCHARGE PLANNING FOR HOME HEALTH CARE
Copyright © 1994, Aspen Publishers, Inc.

National Institute on Deafness and Other Communication Disorders	Information Office 9000 Rockville Pike Bethesda, MD 20892 (301) 496-5751	Research on deafness and communication disorders
National Institute on Dental Research	Information Office Building 31, Room 2C35 9000 Rockville Pike Bethesda, MD 20892 (301) 496-4261	Research on diseases of the mouth and teeth
National Institute on Diabetes and Digestive and Kidney Diseases	Information Office Building 31, Room 9A06 9000 Rockville Pike Bethesda, MD 20892 (301) 496-3583	Research on diabetes mellitus, diseases of the digestive system, and kidney diseases
National Institute on Drug Abuse	Information Office Room 10A46 5600 Fisher Lane Rockville, MD 20857 (301) 443-6500	Research on narcotic addiction and drug abuse
National Institute on Mental Health	Public Inquiries Office Room 15C-05 5600 Fisher Lane Rockville, MD 20857 (301) 443-4513	Research on causes, prevention, and treatment of mental and emotional illnesses
National Institute on Neurological Disorders and Stroke	Information Office Building 31, Room 8A06 9000 Rockville Pike Bethesda, MD 20892 (301) 496-5751	Research on causes, prevention, diagnosis, and treatment of neurological diseases and stroke
National Interfaith Coalition on Aging	P.O. Box 1924 Athens, GA 30603 (404) 353-1331	Research on aging and advice to religious groups that serve the elderly

Discharge Planning for Home Health Care
Copyright © 1994, Aspen Publishers, Inc.

National Kidney Foundation	30 East 33rd Street New York, NY 10016 (212) 889-2210	Promotes prevention, treatment, and cure of kidney diseases
National Kidney and Urologic Diseases Information Clearinghouse	Box NKUDIC Bethesda, MD 20892 (301) 468-6345	Information about kidney diseases
National League for Nursing	10 Columbus Circle New York, NY 10019-1350 (212) 582-1022	To improve the standards for nursing education, nursing services, and health care delivery
National Multiple Sclerosis Society	205 East 42nd Street New York, NY 10017 (212) 986-3240	Research and information about multiple sclerosis
National Osteoporosis Foundation	Suite 822 1625 Eye Street N.W. Washington, DC 20006 (202) 223-2226	To reduce the incidence of osteoporosis
National Pacific/ Asian Resource Center on Aging	Suite 410 2033 Sixth Avenue Seattle, WA 98121-2524 (206) 448-0313	To improve health and social care delivery to the Pacific/ Asian community
National Rehabilitation Association	633 South Washington Street Alexandria, VA 22314 (703) 836-0850	Promotes rehabilitation of persons with disabilities
National Rehabilitation Information Center	Suite 935 8455 Colesville Road Silver Spring, MD 20910 (301) 588-9284 (voice and TDD)	Promotes information about rehabilitation

DISCHARGE PLANNING FOR HOME HEALTH CARE
Copyright © 1994, Aspen Publishers, Inc.

National Rural Health Care Association	Suite 420 301 East Armour Boulevard Kansas City, MO 64111 (816) 756-3140	Health care problems in rural areas
National Self-Help Clearinghouse	33 West 42nd Street New York, NY 10036 (212) 642-2944	Distributes information about self-help groups
National Senior Citizens Law Center	Suite 400 2025 M Street N.W. Washington, DC 20036 (202) 887-5280	Specializes in legal problems of the elderly
National Shut-In Society	P.O. Box 986 Village Station, NY 10014 (212) 222-7699	Brings comfort and support to the housebound
National Stroke Association	Suite 240 300 East Hampden Avenue Englewood, CO 80110 (303) 762-9922	Information about and support for stroke patients and families
National Urban League	500 East 62nd Street New York, NY 10021 (212) 310-9000	Works to eliminate discrimination and to help the economically and socially disadvantaged
National Women's Health Network	1325 G Street N.W. Washington, DC 20005 (202) 347-1140	Clearinghouse on women's health issues
Office on Smoking and Health	Park Building, Room 1-10 5600 Fisher Lane Rockville, MD 20857 (301) 443-1575	Smoking cessation methods and information about health risks
Older Women's League	Suite 300 730 11th Street N.W. Washington, DC 20001 (202) 783-6686	Issues of middle-aged and older women

Copyright © 1994, Aspen Publishers, Inc.

Organization of Chinese Americans	Suite 926 2025 Eye Street N.W. Washington, DC 20006 (202) 223-5500	Equal opportunity for Americans of Chinese ancestry
Public Utilities Commission	Initial contact to this number for information re: locality (800) 693-7380	Rate issues
Retirement Research Foundation	Suite 214 1300 West Higgins Road Park Ridge, IL 60068 (312) 823-4133	To improve the quality of life for older adults
Robert Wood Johnson Foundation	P.O. Box 2316 Princeton, NJ 08543 (609) 452-8701	Private philanthropic foundation focusing on improving health in America
Self Help for Hard of Hearing People	7800 Wisconsin Avenue Bethesda, MD 20814 (301) 657-2248 (voice) (301) 657-2249 (TDD)	To educate and promote the interests of those with impaired hearing
Simon Foundation	Box 835 Wilmette, IL 60091 (312) 864-3913	Education regarding urinary incontinence
Skin Cancer Foundation	Suite 2402 245 Fifth Avenue New York, NY 10016 (212) 725-5176	Information about skin cancer
Social Security Administration	Office of Public Inquiries 6401 Security Boulevard Baltimore, MD 21235 (301) 594-1234	Responsible for retirement, survivors, and disability programs
United Ostomy Association	Suite 120 36 Executive Park Irvine, CA 92714 (714) 660-8624	Information about ostomies and supportive services

Discharge Planning for Home Health Care
Copyright © 1994, Aspen Publishers, Inc.

United Parkinson Foundation	360 West Superior Street Chicago, IL 60610 (312) 664-2344	Supportive services and research on Parkinson's disease
United Seniors Health Cooperative	Suite 500 1334 G Street N.W. Washington, DC 20005 (202) 393-6222	To improve the quality and to reduce the costs of health care and social services for older adults
United Way of America	701 North Fairfax Street Alexandria, VA 22314 (703) 836-7100	Funding support for local agencies and needs assessments
Veterans Administration	Office of Public Affairs 810 Vermont Avenue N.W. Washington, DC 20420 (202) 233-2843	Benefits to veterans and their dependents
Volunteers of America	3813 North Causeway Boulevard Metairie, LA 70002 (504) 837-2652	Programs and services by volunteers
Worker's Compensation	Initial contact to this number to obtain information re: locality (800) 482-2383	Work-related injury benefits
Young Men's Christian Association	101 North Wacker Drive Chicago, IL 60606 (312) 977-0031	To develop leadership and to promote healthy lifestyles
Young Women's Christian Association	726 Broadway New York, NY 10003 (212) 614-2700	Organization of females older than 12 years who participate in community services

Copyright © 1994, Aspen Publishers, Inc.

◆ Appendix E ◆

Durable Medical Equipment Coverage for Home Care*

Durable Medical Equipment	*Indication*
Alternating pressure mattress	Patients susceptible to decubiti
Aquamatic K-Pad (heating pad)	Heat application is therapeutic
Automatic blood pressure monitor	Home dialysis patients
Bed pan	Bed-confined patients
Bedside rails	For hospital bed for bedridden patients
Cane	Impaired ambulation patients
Commode	Bed- or room-confined patients
Crutches	Impaired ambulation patients
Heat lamp	Heat application is therapeutic
Hospital bed	Bed-confined patient—variation restricted to specific diagnosis
Infusion pump	Medically necessary
Inhalator	Breathing-impaired patients
IPPB (Intermittent Positive Pressure Breathing)	Breathing-impaired patients

*All items must be physician prescribed and deemed medically necessary. Coverage is subject to revised Medicare protocols. Coverage is under Part B (i.e., 80% coverage of approved rate).

DISCHARGE PLANNING FOR HOME HEALTH CARE
Copyright © 1994, Aspen Publishers, Inc.

Jobst pneumatic compressor device	Circulatory impaired or lymphedemic patients
Lamb's wool	Patients highly susceptible to skin breakdown
Mattress	Bed-confined patients
Monitor (glucose)	Insulin-dependent diabetics
Nebulizer	Severely breathing-impaired patients
Oxygen concentrator	Severely breathing-impaired patients
Oxygen humidifier	Severely breathing-impaired patients
Oxygen regulator	Severely breathing-impaired patients
Paraffin bath (portable)	Heat application is therapeutic
Patient lifts	Bed-confined patients in need of periodic movement
Portable oxygen system	Severely breathing-impaired patients
Quad cane	Ambulatory-impaired patients
Rollaround chair	Medically necessary
Sitz bath	Perineal infection
Sphygmomanometer with stethoscope	Home dialysis patients
Suction machine	Medically necessary
TENS (Transcutaneous Electrical Nerve Stimulator)	Medically necessary for pain control
Traction	Orthopedic patients
Trapeze bar	Bed-confined patients
Urinal	Bed-confined patients
Ventilator	Respiratory-paralyzed patients
Walker	Ambulatory-impaired patients
Wheelchair	Medically necessary for mobility

DISCHARGE PLANNING FOR HOME HEALTH CARE
Copyright © 1994, Aspen Publishers, Inc.

◆ Appendix F ◆

Case Study: Congestive Heart Failure Hospital Discharge Planning

John Smith is a 69-year-old man who was brought to the emergency department via ambulance with complaints of crushing left chest pain. His wife followed in her car and was helpful with provision of information. Mr. Smith had a history of congestive heart failure, which was the impetus for his early retirement at age 62. His condition was controlled by the use of medication and a no added salt diet. He took daily walks with his wife at the indoor shopping center. During his walk this morning, he complained of some indigestion but later reported that it had passed. This afternoon, while mowing his grass, he became short of breath and developed chest pain. He was admitted for acute care with the diagnosis of acute myocardial infarction with congestive heart failure.

On the initial day of Mr. Smith's hospitalization, the nurse began to develop a rapport with the patient as she proceeded with her initial nursing assessment. Mrs. Smith then provided much of the information on the patient self-assessment form as her husband rested. The couple reside in a rancher that they built 27 years ago. There are three steps to enter the hourse, but otherwise everything is contained on one floor. The couple have helpful neighbors, three supportive children, and seven grandchildren, one of whom they babysit during the day.

Mrs. Smith became very apprehensive when reading the questions about advance directives. She verbalized a fear that her husband might die. The nurse sat with Mrs. Smith briefly and explained what a heart attack is and the usual treatment regime and answered Mrs. Smith's questions. Mrs. Smith thanked the nurse and appeared calmer.

DISCHARGE PLANNING FOR HOME HEALTH CARE
Copyright © 1994, Aspen Publishers, Inc.

Other members of ABC Healthcare's multidisciplinary discharge planning team also made their initial contacts with the patient. The respiratory therapist stayed with Mr. Smith until he felt more ease of breathing. The physician explained the implications of a heart attack and the plan of treatment. She also explained advance directives and noted the desire not to be resuscitated on the patient's record. The utilization management specialist reviewed the record and noted the expected diagnosis-related group reimbursement length of stay to be 8.1 days.

The next morning, the social worker reviewed the patient's record. After talking with the nurse, he spoke with Mr. Smith. During this initial interview, the social worker discovered that the patient and his family had a supportive relationship, a fact that would be beneficial to the discharge planning process. Mr. Smith verbalized his weakened self-concept that his physical condition might not allow him the independence to which he was accustomed. The social worker provided ongoing counseling throughout the patient's hospitalization. He later contacted the home care coordinator because it was evident after talking with Mrs. Smith that the patient would return home.

The home care coordinator reviewed the patient record and spoke with the Smiths. She explained home care availability and funding provided by Medicare. She discussed community provider agencies and offered the patient a choice. The Smiths were aware that referral to Agency A, the patient's preference, was contingent upon needs at discharge and physician collaboration. The home care coordinator assured the Smiths that she would follow up and stop by in a day or two.

By the fifth day of the hospitalization, Mr. Smith no longer required monitoring and was transferred to a medical unit. His new primary nurse contacted the home care coordinator, stating that the patient's son wanted a phone call. The home care coordinator contacted the patient's son and discovered that he had some reservations about the patient's ability to return home. He stated that babysitting for his sister's active 3-year-old would surely kill his father. Barry was agreeable to attending a family meeting, and the home care coordinator planned to notify him with the time. She discussed this conversation at the patient discharge planning meeting only to find that the Smith's older daughter had contacted the social worker to say that the patient should be told he can no longer babysit for the 3-year-old. It had become obvious to the discharge planning team that family dynamics necessitated a family meeting, and a meeting was scheduled for day 6. Attendees included the physician, wife, three children, primary nurse, social worker, and home care coordinator. The patient was not in attendance because of the stressed situation.

The social worker presided at the family conference as each person had an opportunity to discuss his or her thoughts, concerns, and preferences. The social worker advocated for the patient and explained Mr. Smith's desire to return to an independent state. The physician gave a current condition report and explained the need to decrease the patient's stressors and to avoid the patient's becoming crippled by the fear of future heart attacks.

The discussion culminated in the final plan. Mr. Smith would be discharged in 2 days (day 8) with home nursing and aide follow-up. He would require oxygen for the first few weeks,

DISCHARGE PLANNING FOR HOME HEALTH CARE
Copyright © 1994, Aspen Publishers, Inc.

which the respiratory therapist would arrange. The grandchild would be watched by the Smith's oldest daughter for a minimum of 2 to 3 weeks, allowing the patient a stress-free environment. A reevaluation of the patient's condition would be conducted to determine whether he could resume the child's care. All members of the team were pleased with the resolution of the conflict.

Mr. Smith was agreeable to the final plan and was relieved to know that his granddaughter would be well cared for until he was stronger. The discharge planning team worked rapidly to arrange all necessary services and equipment needs in preparation for the discharge, which was scheduled for day 8, a Sunday.

This case study shows that even in seemingly good situations conflict can arise. Often there is a time lag for the conflict to surface, which can greatly inhibit the effectiveness of discharge planning and can lengthen the hospital stay. Every member of the discharge planning team must work actively toward final plans from day 1 of the hospitalization to avoid delays. The impact of one member not following through in a timely manner can be devastating to the bottom line. The team must function as a team, with each member being responsible for certain portions yet working interdependently.

Mr. Smith went home as planned, and his recovery allowed him to resume his previous activities, including the care of his granddaughter: a happy ending for all.

Discharge Planning for Home Health Care
Copyright © 1994, Aspen Publishers, Inc.

Patient Discharge Instructions

Patient name John Smith **Date** 1/28/93

Address 100 Main Street Accompanied by Alma

Anytown, USA 00000 Relationship wife

Medications	*Dose*	*Times*	*Written Information Given*	
			Yes	*No*
Furosemide	40 mg by mouth	Two once a day	X	
Digoxin	0.25 mg by mouth	Daily	X	
Nitroglycerin	grains 1/150 under the tongue	If needed for chest pain	X	

Diet No added salt

Fluid requirements Limit to 2 quarts per day

Personalized instructions

Do not babysit for your grandchild until Dr. Brown authorizes. Remember that this is a stressor.

Decrease all stressors. Rest frequently, and stop activity if you have any chest, neck, jaw, or arm pain, nausea, vomiting, fatigue, lightheadedness, or palpitations.

Next physician visit

Dr. Brown Appt. Feb 3 Ph. 555-1111

Dr.__________ Appt.__________ Ph.__________

Dr.__________ Appt.__________ Ph.__________

Referrals made to

Agency ABC Healthcare Phone 555-0000

Agency will contact patient by ____phone ____writing ✓ patient home visit

Agency__________ Phone__________

Agency will contact patient by ____phone ____writing ____patient home visit

The following valuables were returned: 1 band (yellow metal), 1 wallet, $15

I received a written copy of my discharge instructions after a verbal explanation. I understand these instructions.

____________________ ____________________

Patient/designee Relationship

____

Date

DISCHARGE PLANNING FOR HOME HEALTH CARE
Copyright © 1994, Aspen Publishers, Inc.

◆ Appendix G ◆

Diagnosis-Related Group Discharge Plan, Congestive Heart Failure

(Average Length of Stay, 6.1 Days)

Day	*Discharge Planning Team Member*	*Care*
1	Physician	Admission to hospital: • history/physical • initiate acute care to stabilize patient • relay family/patient dynamics to nurse • address preliminary discharge plan in record
	Nurse	Complete initial nursing assessment Assist with completion of patient self-assessment Refer to social services/home care coordinator
2	Patient	Provide necessary information to discharge planning team
	Family	Provide information about support system to team
	Social worker	Initial patient assessment of psychosocial and postdischarge needs Discuss available community resources

Copyright © 1994, Aspen Publishers, Inc.

Day	*Discharge Planning Team Member*	*Care*
	Home care coordinator	Review record Initiate referral form Discuss home care with patient: • offer choice of provider • explain financial coverage • document patient choice
	Physician	Refine medical treatment
	Respiratory therapist	Begin oxygen instructions in anticipation of postdischarge needs
	Nurse	Begin instruction about congestive heart failure Develop rapport with patient
	Utilization management	Review record, classify patient Notify physician of deficient documentation
3	Physician	Refine medical treatment
	Social worker	Arrange family meeting if necessary
	Dietitian	Begin dietary instruction Provide written diet plan
	Home care coordinator	Elicit physician feedback regarding home care plan
4	Family	Meet with appropriate members of discharge planning team as scheduled Outline support system availability, probable needs Ask questions of team members Follow up as requested
	Social worker	Family conference Make needed referrals (e.g., Meals on Wheels, hospital bed) Document in patient record
	Respiratory therapist	Family conference Obtain orders for arterial blood gases Continue instruction to patient about oxygen and support system Document in patient record
	Dietitian	Family conference Instruct in support system for dietary needs Elicit feedback from patient and reinstruct Document in patient record

DISCHARGE PLANNING FOR HOME HEALTH CARE
Copyright © 1994, Aspen Publishers, Inc.

Day	*Discharge Planning Team Member*	*Care*
	Nurse	Family conference
		Continue to instruct patient about disease process, including when to notify physician
		Document in patient record
	Home care coordinator	Family conference
		Update referral work sheet
		Order needed supplies (e.g., Duoderm for decubitus)
		Document in patient record
	Physician	Refine medication and treatment regime
		Family conference
		Alert entire team of projected discharge date
	Patient	Family conference (if indicated)
		Review educational material
		Relay anticipated problems to discharge planning team
5	Physician	Discharge patient if condition stable
		Document specific treatment regime in record
		Order specific home care and sign referral
		Order oxygen if needed
		Communicate need for follow-up to patient and nurse
	Respiratory therapist	Refer for home oxygen, provide oxygen company with arterial blood gas levels
		Continue oxygen instructions with patient
		Document actions in patient record
	Nurse	Prepare written discharge instructions
		Review instructions with patient and family, if indicated: • elicit feedback to ascertain level of understanding • reinstruct if necessary • document on patient instruction checklist
	Home care coordinator	Answer any last-minute patient/family questions
		Refer care to provider of patient's preference
		Assess completion and accuracy of referral and work sheet
		Forward referral and work sheet to provider agency

Discharge Planning for Home Health Care
Copyright © 1994, Aspen Publishers, Inc.

Day	Discharge Planning Team Member	Care
	Dietitian	Elicit feedback and answer questions
	Patient	Ask any/all questions
	Family	Take patient home
	Utilization management	Review record for diagnosis-related group information
	Finance	Discuss payment expectations and plans with patient before discharge

Discharge Planning for Home Health Care
Copyright © 1994, Aspen Publishers, Inc.

◆ Appendix H ◆

Case Study: Diabetes Mellitus

John Doe is a 66-year-old retired carpenter who lives in a self-built mountain cabin with his wife. His three married children live within 20 miles. John's medical history is unremarkable. He is 6 ft 2 in tall and weighs 190 lb, 20 lb less than 6 months ago.

John was admitted to Hospital A after complaints of excessive thirst with frequent urination. His sleep was interrupted five to six times per night because of urinary frequency. He describes his activity level as sluggish and states that he isn't "up to par."

John's fasting blood sugar (FBS) was 436 mg/dl (milligrams per deciliter). He was diagnosed with juvenile type diabetes, and his symptoms subsided with the use of insulin NPH. He and his wife had no prior knowledge of diabetes or its treatment. Both were interested in learning everything there was to learn but had some difficulty learning insulin administration.

PSYCHOSOCIAL STATUS

John is alert and oriented. He and his wife have a good relationship and enjoy outdoor activities together. Both are somewhat anxious about John's new diagnosis yet are eager to learn.

DISCHARGE PLANNING FOR HOME HEALTH CARE
Copyright © 1994, Aspen Publishers, Inc.

SYSTEM REVIEW

- *Cardiovascular*—apical pulse: 88; blood pressure: R arm 132/80, L arm 128/76; heart sounds: regular; no noted edema
- *Pulmonary*—all lung fields clear; 22 breath/min; tissue perfusion indicates good oxygenation
- *Neurological*—PEARL; oriented × 3; reflexes good; no tremors
- *Gastrointestinal*—active bowel sounds; abdomen soft; 20-lb weight loss past 6 months; last b.m. yesterday; fruity breath
- *Musculoskeletal*—range of motion all joints within normal limits; progressive fatigue, requires increased amounts of sleep
- *Genitourinary*—nocturia × 6; urine clear
- *Integumentary*—unremarkable

DIAGNOSIS

Adult onset juvenile diabetes

MEDICATIONS

Insulin NPH, 24 u subcutaneously each day.

HOSPITALIZATION SUMMARY

- Day 1
  - —Admitted
  - —Nursing assessment
  - —Medical history and physical
  - —Completion of initial lab work
- Day 2
  - —FBS 436 mg/dl (milligrams per deciliter)
  - —Initiation of insulin therapy
  - —Patient education re: condition, treatment started
  - —Referral made for dietary consult
- Day 3
  - —FBS 360 mg/dl (milligrams per deciliter)
  - —Insulin dose adjustment made
  - —Continuation of patient education with wife present:
    1. Wife resistant to performing insulin injection
    2. Patient prepared syringe with many verbal cues
    3. Practice session with normal saline; return demonstration of prefilling by patient and wife

DISCHARGE PLANNING FOR HOME HEALTH CARE
Copyright © 1994, Aspen Publishers, Inc.

- —Dietary consult: written/verbal instructions re: 1,800-cal American Diabetes Association (ADA) diet provided to patient and wife
- —Social service consult completed
- —Home health consult completed

- Day 4
  - —FBS 180 mg/dl (milligrams per deciliter)
  - —Insulin dose adjustment made
  - —Continuation of patient education:
    1. Patient prefilled syringe independently and self-injected with verbal cues
    2. Dietary recall obtained and dietary reinstruction provided
    3. Patient and wife reinstructed about signs and symptoms of hypoglycemia and hyperglycemia
- Day 5
  - —FBS 118 mg/dl (milligrams per deciliter)
  - —Continuation of patient education:
    1. Patient prefilled syringe and self-injected independently; no verbal cues required
    2. Wife prefilled syringe independently and demonstrated injection techniques on an orange
    3. Patient and wife provided appropriate recall regarding 1,800-cal American Diabetes Association (ADA) diet
    4. Patient and wife recalled limited information about hypoglycemia and hyperglycemia
  - —Patient discharged with follow-up home care referral
    1. Diagnosis-related group length of stay: 5.9 days ($2,463.58)
    2. Length of stay: 5.0 days
    3. Savings: 0.9 days (approximately $500.00)

HOME CARE SUMMARY

- Day 1
  - —FBS 122 mgm/dl (milligrams per deciliter)
  - —Patient admitted for skilled nursing services
  - —Continuation of patient instructions:
    1. Patient provided second independent return demonstration of insulin self-administration
    2. Written materials provided with emphasis on teaching function of pancreas, effects of insulin, and signs/symptoms of hypoglycemia and hyperglycemia
    3. Observation of wife's injection technique on orange
    4. Patient to keep food diary
- Day 2
  - —FBS 116 mgm/dl (milligrams per deciliter)

Copyright © 1994, Aspen Publishers, Inc.

- —Wife provided insulin administration, required verbal cues for injection
- —Continuation of patient instructions, especially of disease process:
  1. Partial recall of information with reinstruction regarding disease process
  2. Food diary evaluated with instructions on need for modifications
  3. Patient and wife planned to read all education material in preparation for tomorrow's visit
- Day 3
  - —FBS 118 mg/dl (milligrams per deciliter)
  - —Wife provided independent return demonstration of insulin administration
  - —Patient and wife recalled disease process and diet appropriateness
  - —Patient and wife provided with phone numbers for ADA
  - —Physician notified of status
  - —Patient discharged from skilled home care follow-up

Follow-up contact in 1 week revealed that John had returned to his outdoor activities. He denied feelings of fatigue and reported that a recent FBS remained stable. He was appreciative of the coordination of care between the hospital and the home care provider. He plans to tell all his friends about the well-coordinated and high-quality care he received.

DISCHARGE PLANNING FOR HOME HEALTH CARE
Copyright © 1994, Aspen Publishers, Inc.

◆ Appendix I ◆

Hospital Clinical Pathway: Diabetes Mellitus

Assigned Case Manager:________________

Activity	*Preadmission*	*Admission* Day 1	Day 2	Day 3	Day 4	Day 5
Testing						
Laboratory	FBS	FBS, electrolytes, complete blood count	FBS	FBS	FBS	FBS
Radiology		Chest radiograph				
Cardiac		ECG				
Respiratory						
Other						
Preadmission consults						
Cardiac						
Specialty	Endocrinologist	N/A	N/A	N/A	N/A	N/A
Inpatient consults						
Dietary			Dietitian			
Specialty						
Other		Nursing assessment, H&P		Social service home care		
Diet	1,800-cal ADA	1,800-cal ADA	1,800-cal ADA	1,800-cal ADA	1,800-cal ADA	1,800-cal ADA
Treatments						
Medications			Insulin NPH, 24 U s.q. q A.M.	Insulin NPH, 30 U s.q. q A.M.	Insulin NPH, 30 U s.q. q A.M.	Insulin NPH, 30 U s.q. q A.M. D/C'd
Discharge planning		Nursing assessment	Discussion at D/C plan meeting	Social service and home care assessment	Family meeting	
Education		Disease process	1,800-cal ADA diet, treatment, insulin administration	Insulin administration; return demo; return feedback re: diet, S/S of hypo--glycemia	Insulin return demo; return feedback re: S/S of hyperglycemia	Prevention D/C instructions

Copyright © 1994, Aspen Publishers, Inc.

◆ Appendix J ◆

Home Health Clinical Pathway: Diabetes Mellitus

Assigned Case Manager:______________________

Activity	*Visit 1*	*Visit 2*	*Visit 3*	*Visit 4*
Direct care Assessment	Physical assessment Vital signs, subjective data, side effects of medications	FBS, vital signs, subjective data, side effects of medications	FBS, vital signs, subjective data, side effects of medications	N/A
Referrals	Aide care p.r.n.			N/A
Education Medications	Medication regime, route, and scheduling; return feedback re: route and schedule; verbal insulin administration instruction	Return demo of insulin administration with verbal cues	Return demo of insulin administration (independent)	N/A
Disease process	S/S hypoglycemia, Rx for hypoglycemia, when to call the physician	Return feedback re: hypoglycemia, S/S hyperglycemia, Rx for hyperglycemia	Return feedback re: hyperglycemia, when to visit the physician	
Discharge planning	Discussion of home care plan of care, including time of discharge	Planning with support system	D/C (instructions provided)	N/A

DISCHARGE PLANNING FOR HOME HEALTH CARE
Copyright © 1994, Aspen Publishers, Inc.

◆ Appendix K ◆

Hospital Clinical Pathway: Congestive Heart Failure

Assigned Case Manager:____________________

		Admission			
Activity	*Preadmission*	*Day 1*	*Day 2*	*Day 3*	*Day 4*
Testing					
Laboratory	N/A	Electrolytes, complete blood count	Electrolytes	Electrolytes	Electrolytes
Radiology	N/A	Chest radiograph			
Cardiac	N/A	ECG			Chest radiograph
Respiratory	N/A	Pulmonary function test			ECG
Other	N/A				
Preadmission consults					
Cardiac	N/A				
Specialty	N/A				
Inpatient consults					
Dietary	N/A	Consult made	Patient instruct in NAS diet	Patient feedback	
Specialty	N/A	Cardiac disease process	Cardiac prevention	Cardiac treatment	Cardiac medications, when to call the physician
Other	N/A	Respiratory use of O_2		Respiratory (deep-breathing exercises)	
Diet	N/A	NAS	NAS	NAS	NAS
Treatments	N/A	IV Bumex, spirometry	IV Bumex, spirometry	p.o. Bumex, spirometry	p.o. Bumex, spirometry
Medications	N/A	IV Bumex, Lanoxin	IV Bumex, Lanoxin	p.o. Bumex, Lanoxin	p.o. Bumex, Lanoxin
D/C planning	N/A	Intake information	Patient interview	Family meeting, physician collaboration	Discharge
Education	N/A	Disease process, oxygen use	NAS diet, prevention of acute episodes	Treatment, deep-breathing exercises	Medications

Discharge Planning for Home Health Care
Copyright © 1994, Aspen Publishers, Inc.

◆ Appendix L ◆

Home Health Clinical Pathway: Acute Exacerbation of Congestive Heart Failure

Assigned Case Manager:__________________

Activity	*Visit 1*	*Visit 2*	*Visit 3*	*Visit 4*	*Visit 5*
Direct care	Physical assessment	Electrolytes			Electrolytes
Assessment	BP T/P/R Lung sounds Edema levels JVD Home safety Support system Weight	BP T/P/R Lung sounds Edema levels JVD Home safety Support system Weight	BP T/P/R Lung sounds Edema levels JVD Home safety Support system Weight	BP T/P/R Lung sounds Edema levels JVD Home safety Support system Weight	BP T/P/R Lung sounds Edema levels JVD Home safety Support system Weight
Referrals	HME company p.r.n. Aide care Area Agency on Aging		Physician update		AHA
Education	Medication route and schedule	Medication action/ SE #1	Return feed-back re: medication, action/SE #1, action/SE #2	Return feed-back re: medication, action/SE #2, action/SE #3	Return feedback re: medication, action/SE #3, action/SE #4
Disease process	When to call physician	Disease process	Preventive measures	Treatment	Community agency support
D/C planning	Discussion of home care plan of care, including time of D/C	Adaptation of current environ-ment	Planning with support system for future		

DISCHARGE PLANNING FOR HOME HEALTH CARE
Copyright © 1994, Aspen Publishers, Inc.

Bibliography

Abramson, J. Enhancing patient participation: Clinical strategies in the discharge planning process. *Social Work in Health Care.* 1990; 14:53–71.

Accreditation manual for hospitals. (1992). Oakbrook Terrace, IL: Joint Commission on Accreditation of Healthcare Organizations.

A profile of the home care community. *NAHC.* 1988; Fact sheet #1.

Callendar, J. Discharge planning, a critical role. *HSN Program Guide.* 1991; January:4–6.

Corkery, E. Discharge planning and home health care: What every staff nurse should know. *Orthopedic Nursing.* 1989; 8:18–27.

Crittendon, F.J. (1983). *Discharge planning for health care facilities.* Los Angeles, CA: Allied Health Publications.

Curtin, L., & Surlage, C. (1984). *DRG's: The reorganization of health.* Chicago, IL: SN Publications.

DRG study shows disparity among hospitals. *Modern Health Care.* 1991; January 28:18.

Evans, R.L., et al. Timing of social work intervention and medical patients length of hospital stay. *Health and Social Work Report.* 1989;277–282.

Feldstein, P.J. (1988). *Health Care Economics.* New York, NY: Wiley & Sons.

Frasca, C., & Cristy, M.W. Assuring continuity of care through a hospital based home health agency. *QRB.* 1986; May:167–171.

Gingerich, B. (1987). *Position paper on multidisciplinary discharge planning.* Glassrock.

Hartigan, E.G., & Brown, D.J. (1977). *Discharge planning for continuity of care.* New York, NY: National League for Nursing.

Hawkes, J. Hospital costs below average here. *The Intelligencer Journal.* 1991; 35,580:A1–A2.

Health Care Financing Administration. (1993). *Home care statistics.* Washington, DC: NAHC.

HCFA considers gradual approach to outpatient payment reform. *Hospitals.* 1991; May: 30–33.

Johnson, E., & Jackson, J. Teaching the home care client. *Nursing Clinics of North America.* 1989; 24:687–692.

Joint Commission on Accreditation of Healthcare Organizations. (1993). *Standards for the Accreditation of home care.* Oakbrook Terrace, IL: Joint Commission on Accreditation of Healthcare Organizations.

Koontz, O., & Welrich, D. (1984). *Management.* 8th ed. New York, NY: McGraw-Hill.

Landry, E. (1990). *The complete Medicare handbook.* Rocklin, CA: Prima Publishing and Communication.

Lewin, K. (1951). *Field Theory in Social Sciences.* New York, NY: Harper & Row.

Luken, P. Hospital based discharge planning. The beginning of home care for many. *Caring.* 1991; X:18–23.

McCay, E., et al. (1990). *Factors influencing patients' informational needs at time of discharge.* New York, NY: Elsevier Scientific Publishers.

McClelland, E., et al. (1985). *Continuity of care: Advancing the concept of discharge planning.* San Diego, CA: Grune & Stratton.

McKeehan, K., et al. (1981). *Continuity of care, a multidisciplinary approach to discharge planning.* St. Louis, MO: Mosby.

Patient discharge and referral planning—Whose responsibility? (1974). New York, NY: Council of Hospital and Related Institutional Nursing Services.

Proper discharge policies can help you avoid liability. *Hospital Home Health.* 1988; 5:61–64.

Quality Assurance in home care and hospice organizations. (1990). Oakbrook, IL: Joint Commission on Accreditation of Healthcare Organizations.

Rorden, J.W., & Taft, E. (1990). *Discharge planning guide for nurses.* Philadelphia, PA: Saunders.

Rubin, I.M., et al. (1978). *Managing human resources in health care organizations.* Reston, VA: Reston Publishing.

Russ, G.W. (1986). *Discharge planning, policy and procedure guideline manual.* Los Angeles, CA: Academy Medical Systems.

Sandrick, K. RBRVS impact. *Hospitals.* 1992; 66(24):14–15.

Simpson, J.E.P., & Levitt, R. (1981). *Going home.* New York, NY: Churchill Livingstone.

Smith, J.B. Effective discharge planning and home health care. How to's for the staff nurse. *Advancing Clinical Care.* 1990; 1:6–8.

Stand up and cheer. (editorial). *Health and Social Work.* 1989; 11:227–230.

Stauffer, C. Hospital costs here below average. *Lancaster New Era.* 1991:35,580:B1–B2.

Steffl, B.M., & Eide, I. (1978). *Discharge planning handbook.* Thorofare, NJ: Slack.

The crises in home health care: Greater need, less care. (1986). Report to the Senate Special Committee on Aging.

Thliveris, M. A hospital wide discharge planning program. *Dimensions.* 1990(February).

Waldo, D., et al. National health expenditures 1985. *Health Care Financing Review.* 1985; 8:16.

Wimberly, E., and Blazyk, S. Monitoring patient outcome following discharge: A computerized geriatric case management system. *Health and Social Work.* 1989; 14:269.

Yate, M. (1990). *Hiring the best.* Holbrook, MA: Perigne McCoy.

Zarle, N.C. (1987). *Continuing care, the process and practice of discharge planning.* Gaithersburg, MD: Aspen Publishers.

INSERT

TAB

◆ Index ◆

A

Note: Page numbers in *italics* denote figures and exhibits; those followed by "t" denote tables.

B

C

D

I

J

K

L

M

N

O

P

Q

R

S

T

U

V

W

Y

9 780834 205727

Printed in Dunstable, United Kingdom

88190709R00152